Medical Receptionists and Secretaries Handbook

Fourth edition

Mari Robbins

Radcliffe Publishing
Oxford • Seattle

Radcliffe Publishing Ltd
18 Marcham Road
Abingdon
Oxon OX14 1AA
United Kingdom

www.radcliffe-oxford.com
Electronic catalogue and worldwide online ordering facility.

First edition 1996
Second edition 1998
Third edition 2002

British Library Cataloguing in Publication Data

A catalogue record for this book is available from the British Library.

ISBN-10 1 85775 726 2
ISBN-13 978 1 85775 726 2

Typeset by AMA DataSet Limited, Preston, Lancs
Printed and bound by TJ International Ltd, Padstow, Cornwall

Contents

Preface

Once again, I am delighted to have the opportunity to revise the *Medical Receptionists and Secretaries Handbook* in readiness for the publication of its fourth edition.

The continued escalation of changes in the National Health Service since 2001 has given me the challenge of a continually changing situation! However, I have endeavoured to ensure that the information contained in this edition is as up to date as possible.

More and more reforms, quality issues and advances in information technology mean that health service managers as well as healthcare professionals rely on the support of receptionists and secretaries working as a team in healthcare provision to give an efficient, high-quality service to both patients and the public.

These are times of continuing change for **all** involved in the provision and delivery of healthcare, based on identified patient needs, whether working in the NHS, social care or the private sector. It is therefore vital that they have a knowledge and understanding of what these changes involve.

I cannot over-emphasise the important role of the medical receptionist and secretary in providing the vital link between patients and healthcare professionals in the NHS and private sectors.

Mari Robbins
January 2006

Contributors

Sally Storey
Director of Human Resources and Organisational Development
Queen Elizabeth Hospital NHS Trust
Woolwich
London

Roy Lilley
Former Trust Chairman
Writer and broadcaster on NHS Issues

Acknowledgements

My acknowledgements go to Ivan Chu (Health and Safety Adviser, Bournewood Community and Mental Health Trust), Sue Dunlop (Secretary to Professor J Cobb and Mr G Etherington, Harley Street, London), Marjorie Lear (Practice Manager, Oxshott Medical Centre, Surrey) and Barbara Stewart (Pharmacist, West Sussex).

In revising material for this edition, I have found both the NHS and the Department of Health websites an invaluable source of current information.

The National Health Service

History

Prior to the National Health Service Act of 1946, healthcare in the UK had developed in an ad hoc manner.

The medical profession had, since the latter part of the nineteenth century, gradually acquired social respectability, legal status and economic strength. The concept of public responsibility for the health of individuals can be traced back to 1834, when the Poor Law Amendment Act was passed, which established that parish workhouses should provide sick wards where the able-bodied inhabitants could be treated when they became unwell. However, as the health of the community had been severely neglected, it became necessary for the workhouses to admit the sick paupers from the parish to their wards – people who had hitherto been left to die as they were unable to obtain medical care themselves. By 1848 the demand for institutional care was such that the sick wards of the workhouses had become entirely devoted to sick paupers. The Public Health Act of that year acknowledged for the first time the State's responsibility for institutional care.

The quality of medical care available improved as scientists made important discoveries. Florence Nightingale, in her contribution to both nurse training and hospital planning, revolutionised the standards of institutional care. Largely due to the philanthropy of the well-to-do and the moral obligations of the charitable and religious bodies, the end of the nineteenth century heralded the opening of many voluntary and private hospitals. Voluntary hospitals were financed through subscriptions and donations, and attracted the services of skilled doctors, some of whom, acting on their social conscience, often treated patients without payment.

The beginning of the twentieth century saw the advent of insurance schemes which enabled individuals to protect themselves against sickness and injuries which might involve them in expensive medical care or affect their capacity to work.

However, despite the progress that was being made, the standard of medical and nursing care emerging throughout the country was inconsistent in both quality and availability.

At the end of the First World War, the first Ministry of Health was established, which together with various reforms provided the stimulus for a nationally organised health service. The Second World War brought about further reforms and the publishing of the Beveridge Report in 1942 with its recommendations that formed the basis for the post-war system of social welfare services, and the provision of a comprehensive system of healthcare. Sir William Beveridge recommended that the term 'comprehensive' meant that medical treatment should be available for every citizen, both in the home and in hospital, and provided by general practitioners, specialist physicians and surgeons, dentists, opticians, nurses and midwives. He also advocated the provision of surgical appliances and rehabilitation services.

Thus the National Health Service (NHS) became effective in 1948, with the aim of improving the health of the people, providing healthcare through a system of public finance and public provision and, by eradicating disease, reducing the demand for free healthcare services. The NHS took over all hospitals, convalescent homes and rehabilitation units, offering consultants contracts as full-time salaried employees. General medical practitioners providing family doctor services were encouraged to sign contracts to provide family practitioner services for patients in their area, and were permitted to remain self-employed but paid by the health service on a fee basis.

Medical services fell into the following three functional areas:

- those concerned with the sick person in the community
- those concerned with the sick person in an institution
- those concerned with preventive medical services.

They were identified with the following services:

- general practitioner services
- hospital services
- services provided by the local authority (excluding school health services).

The hospital service was administered by regional hospital boards, which absorbed all of the public and voluntary hospitals in the country. The national planning of hospital requirements was established.

Teaching hospitals in England and Wales remained relatively independent with their boards of governors who were responsible directly to the

Secretary of State, but they were linked only to the regional hospital boards in that there was one teaching hospital in each region.

General practitioner services were organised through executive councils, which administered the family doctors' contracts and dental, pharmaceutical and ophthalmic services. The local health authorities administered the preventive services, ambulance services, etc.

The main advantage of the NHS was that it had brought together services which had previously been under the control of independent organisations. However, administration of this tripartite arrangement was far from satisfactory, and in an attempt to improve the co-ordination of healthcare between hospital boards, local executive councils and the type of care provided by local authorities, the 1974 National Health Service Reorganisation Act came into force.

Reorganising the NHS

The 1974 reorganisation brought about major changes in the way in which the NHS was organised and structured.

The changes introduced to the NHS the concept of planning and improvement in personnel and manpower controls.

One issue that arose from this reorganisation and which remains today was the creation of the Health Service Commissioner role.

Health Service Commissioner (Ombudsman)

The Health Service Commissioner (Ombudsman) undertakes independent investigation into complaints about the NHS, as well as Government departments and other public bodies. It is completely independent of the NHS and the Government. In the NHS the Ombudsman investigates complaints that a hardship or injustice has been caused by its failure to provide a service either as a result of a failure in service or due to mis-administration. The Ombudsman also looks into complaints against private health providers, but only if the treatment was funded by the NHS.

Complainants can only refer their cases to the Ombudsman after failing to achieve a resolution with the organisation or practitioner they are complaining against – for example, because of delays in dealing with a complaint locally or failure to obtain a satisfactory answer to a complaint. The Ombudsman can consider complaints from a patient, a close member of the family, or a partner or representative if the patient is unable to act for him- or herself, or from someone who has suffered injustice or hardship as a result of the actions of the NHS. A complaint will normally only be considered within a year of the events which gave rise to it.

The Ombudsman publishes detailed reports of investigations which identify common themes in complaints. The reports are intended to be used as training tools to improve services, and chief executives are asked to ensure that all clinical directors and complaints managers are made aware of them. They are also considered by the House of Commons public administration committee.

Further information can be found at www.ombudsman.org.uk

The 1982 reorganisation

The 1982 reorganisation aimed to simplify the health service and deliver greater efficiency and accountability of the service to Parliament. It also aimed to strengthen local-level management.

The NHS

The NHS is now the largest organisation in Europe, and is recognised as one of the best health services in the world by the World Health Organization, but there need to be improvements to cope with the demands of the twenty-first century.

The NHS is mainly financed through taxation, and therefore relies on Parliament for funding, and is accountable to Parliament through the Secretary of State for Health. Parliamentary procedures ensure that the Government has to publicly explain and defend its policies for the NHS.

The NHS is changing the way in which it works in order to ensure that patients always come first. Figure 1.2 indicates how the new structure works in England, and details of the health service in other parts of the UK can be found at www.nhsuk/Wales(Scotland/NorthernIreland:)

Department of Health (DH)

This is the department that supports the Government in improving the health and well-being of the population. It is responsible for:

• the NHS

• social services

• public health.

The DH negotiates levels of NHS funding with the Treasury and allocates resources to the health service.

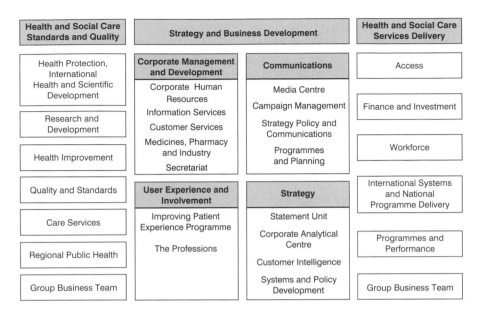

Figure 1.1 Structure of the Department of Health.

It can be seen from Figure 1.1, which demonstrates the present structure of the DH, that it is divided into three groups:

- health and social care standards and quality
- strategy and business development
- delivery of health and social care.

The DH is currently involved in an 18-month programme of change that will reduce (or transfer) its staff by nearly 40%. Some posts will be abolished and others will be transferred to other national bodies. This demonstrates the Government's policy of shifting power from Whitehall to frontline healthcare personnel. The new role of the DH will be to provide strategic leadership to NHS and social care organisations by, for example:

- setting the overall direction
- ensuring that national standards are set
- securing resources
- making major investment decisions
- driving choice for patients and users.

Structure of the NHS

Special health authorities

Special health authorities provide a service to England rather than to individual local communities. Although independent, they can be subject to ministerial direction in the same way as other health bodies. There are currently 19 special health authorities, including the following:

- Mental Health Act Commission

- National Blood Authority

- Prescription Pricing Authority

- UK Transplant Support Service Authority.

Special health authorities are part of the stand-alone national organisations and are one of the arm's-length bodies (ALBs).

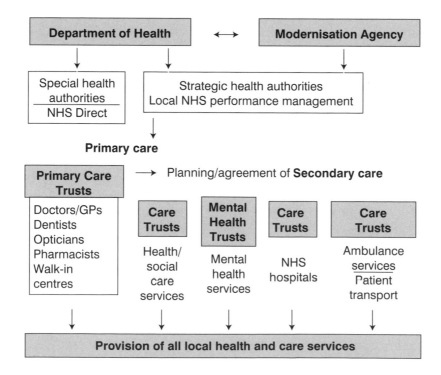

Figure 1.2   Structure of the NHS.

Arm's-length bodies

Arm's-length bodies are stand-alone national organisations which have executive functions and are sponsored by the DH. They have boards, employ staff and publish accounts. They also include non-departmental public bodies, which are set up when independent advice is required without direct influence from Whitehall. There are three categories of arm's-length bodies:

1   *commissions*, which have a role in national government but are not part of any department

2   *advisory bodies*, which assist with evaluating, investigating and supporting policy development in key areas

3   *tribunals*, which are created by legislation and make decisions in specialised fields of law.

Arm's-length bodies are accountable to the DH and in some cases directly to Parliament. They have existed since the NHS came into force in 1948, and by 2004 there were 34 arm's-length bodies, but it has been announced by the Government that their number will be cut to 20 by 2008. Their roles will include the following:

• regulation

• standards

• public welfare

• central services to the NHS.

Shifting the balance of power within the NHS

Two documents – *Securing Delivery* (published in July 2001) and *The Next Steps* (published in January 2002) – outlined the rationale behind devolving power from the Government to frontline NHS organisations, especially primary care trusts. They pointed out that strategic health authorities (SHAs) were to replace the existing 95 health authorities, and that the DH would have a reduced role in directly managing the NHS.

Strategic health authorities

Strategic health authorities (of which there are 28 in total) manage the NHS locally on behalf of the DH, each covering a population of 1.8 million. They have three key functions:

1   Avon, Gloucestershire and
    Wiltshire
2   Bedfordshire and
    Hertfordshire
3   Birmingham and the
    Black Country
4   Cheshire and Merseyside
5   County Durham and Tees
    Valley
6   Coventry, Warwickshire,
    Herefordshire and
    Worcestershire
7   Cumbria and Lancashire
8   Essex
9   Greater Manchester
10 Hampshire and
    Isle of Wight
11 Kent and Medway
12 Leicestershire,
    Northamptonshire
    and Rutland

13 Norfolk, Suffolk and Cambridgeshire
14 North and East Yorkshire and
    Northern Lincolnshire
15 North Central London
16 North East London
17 North West London
18 Northumberland, Tyne and Wear
19 Shropshire and Staffordshire
20 Somerset and Dorset

21 South East London
22 South West London
23 South West Peninsula
24 South Yorkshire
25 Surrey and Sussex
26 Thames Valley
27 Trent
28 West Yorkshire

Figure 1.3   Strategic health authority areas.

- creating a coherent strategic framework
- agreeing annual performance targets of primary care trusts and NHS trusts
- building capacity and supporting performance improvement.

They develop strategies for capital investment, information management and development of the workforce, and they arbitrate and/or solve any problems or conflict that may arise between local NHS organisations. They also foster partnerships with non-NHS bodies, universities and further education institutions, and they help local authorities' overview and scrutiny committees to monitor the health service. SHAs ensure that there is consultation about major service reconfigurations.

Primary care trusts

Primary care trusts (PCTs) run primary and community services on a local basis and commission secondary care, and are considered to be the 'cornerstone' of the NHS locally. There are 302 PCTs, each serving an average population of approximately 170 000. The Government has stated that the health service should be primary care led, especially since primary care staff are well placed to have an overview of hospital and community services, of public health and health services, and of local authorities and the NHS. Please see Chapter 12 for more detailed information.

NHS trusts

There are three main types of NHS trust:

- 176 acute trusts, which provide both medical and surgical care, usually centred on a teaching or district general hospital (an acute trust may manage more than one hospital)
- 88 trusts that provide mental health services both in the community and in hospital
- 31 ambulance trusts.

Some trusts may manage only specialist facilities (e.g. eye or dental hospitals), while others may manage a combination of the above services.

By providing healthcare commissioned by PCTs, and set out in the service-level agreement between the two organisations, NHS trusts earn their income. They have a legal duty to break even financially, and they earn a 6% return on their capital. NHS trusts must work in partnership with other NHS organisations, local authorities and voluntary sectors, and they must deliver national priorities.

Foundation trusts

Foundation trusts were created in order to give greater freedom to NHS organisations by moving from a service that is controlled nationally to one in which standards and inspection are national, but delivery and account-ability are locally monitored. Foundation trust status is subject to the trust's standards, performance ratings and inspection systems. Although foundation trusts are accountable to Parliament, staff, patients and the local community have a say in the running of them by becoming 'members' or governors.

Monitor is the independent regulator of NHS foundation trusts. It authorises NHS trusts applying for foundation trust status, and ensures that they comply with the terms of the authorisation (e.g. an obligation to achieve national targets and standards). *Monitor* is accountable to Parliament.

The main advantages of foundation trusts include increased ability to retain any operating surpluses, not being subject to directions from the Secretary of State, and the ability to vary staff pay over and above nation-ally agreed terms and conditions.

Currently, foundation trust status has been given to the highest-performing NHS trusts. However, the Government has announced that by 2008 all NHS trusts will have the opportunity to become foundation trusts. There are 31 foundation trusts at the time of writing, with a further 32 trusts (including mental health trusts) applying in 2005.

Children's trusts

In 2004, the Government published a Green Paper entitled *Every Child Matters*, which states their intention to incorporate services for children within a single organisation. It is anticipated that by 2006 most areas should have their own children's trust, with a children's services director in overall charge.

Children's trusts may be a single organisation or may integrate with other services (e.g. social care, education and the voluntary sector).

Care trusts

Care trusts are designed to allow the integration of health and social care. They commission and provide both services within a single NHS organisation.

Clinical networks

Receptionists and secretaries should be aware that clinical networks exist which provide partnerships involving all organisations and professionals. They enable liaison between primary, secondary and tertiary care as well as between health and social care. Clinical networks ensure that all staff with whom a patient has contact are working to the same protocols (e.g. on patient admission, discharge and transfer). By integrating all of the information that is relevant to a clinical condition, they enable staff to work together for the benefit of the patient. Clinical networks are well established in cancer care.

Nurse prescribing

The Health and Social Care Bill provides for legislative changes that will not only allow increased nurse prescribing across the UK, but will also extend prescribing rights to other professional groups.

Patient Advocacy and Liaison Services (PALS)

Patient Advocacy and Liaison Services (PALS) were set up in 2002 to replace the Community Health Councils which came into being with the changes in the NHS in 1974. Every primary care trust and NHS trust should have a PALS which provides readily accessible help and information to patients, their families and carers about local health services. The aims of PALS are to:

- resolve the complaints and concerns of patients, their families and carers as quickly as possible before they become major problems
- give advice to people about local support groups, and to facilitate contact with them
- provide information about the complaints procedure and independent complaints advocacy support
- monitor the local health services, highlight any perceived gaps in those services and make reports for action to trust managers.

Delivering the NHS Plan: next steps on investment, next steps to reform

This document, which was published in April 2002, introduced plans to reform the financial flows of the NHS through payment by results, and emphasised patient choice and commitment to promoting diversity of healthcare through joint ventures with the private sector.

The NHS Plan

The NHS Plan is the foundation of the Government's reforms for modernising the health service and links change explicitly to extra investment. The Plan was published in July 2002, and set out an ambitious ten-year programme aiming to tackle systematic problems dating from 1948 when the NHS was formed.

The main features of the NHS Plan can be summarised as follows.

- Funding will continue to come from taxation, with services free at the point of use.

- Facilities will include extra beds and equipment, new hospitals and new primary care centres. There will also be a clean-up campaign for hospitals, improved catering services offering better food, and modernisation of GP premises.

- In terms of staff, there will be more doctors, nurses and therapists, more training places, and better pay and working conditions (including more childcare support).

- In terms of performance standards, there will be core national standards and targets, and independent quality inspection with incentives.

- There will be partnership with social services.

- There will be new contracts for GPs and consultants.

- Nurses will have expanded roles, and there will be the introduction of modern matrons and nurse consultants.

- Patients will be given more information and representation, with increased choice.

- There will be a concordat with the private sector to encourage partnerships.

- Waiting times for GP appointments are to be reduced to a maximum of 48 hours. Accident and Emergency and other waiting times are to be cut.

- A national target is to be introduced for reducing health inequalities, and new screening programmes and smoking cessation services are to be introduced.

- Clinical priorities include a major expansion in cancer screening programmes, rapid access to chest pain clinics, shorter waits for heart operations, and new mental health teams.

Further information can be found at www.dh.gov.uk

A new approach to the health of the public – *Choosing Health: making health choices easier*

England needs a new approach to the health of the public, involving policies and approaches that reflect the realities of people's lives today. This means an approach that respects the freedom of individual choice and addresses the fact that too many people and groups have been ignored in the past, and which moves forward at the pace that people want and will support.

Informed choice

Patients want to be able to make their own decisions about choices that impact on their health, and to be given reliable information to help them to do this. They expect the Government to provide support by helping to create the right environment, but it must be remembered that it is important to exercise a special responsibility for children who are too young to make informed choices themselves. Special arrangements also need to be made for those cases where one person's choice may cause harm or nuisance to another (e.g. exposure to second-hand smoke). Rights and responsibilities must be balanced in ways that protect health.

Personalisation

Some people want support in making healthy choices and keeping to them, particularly in deprived groups and communities where current services do not meet their needs. To tackle health inequalities effectively, support must be tailored to the realities of individual lives, with service and support personalised sensitively and provided flexibly and conveniently.

Working together

Individuals cannot make progress with healthier choices on their own, but rather this depends on effective partnerships across communities, including local government, the NHS, the voluntary sector, the media, communities and many others.

Improving healthcare: the NHS Improvement Plan

Improvements in the quality of care have been achieved through the development of National Service Frameworks and the work of the Healthcare Commission. More treatment and care are now available closer to home, and patient choice has begun to have an impact on the way in which the NHS works.

Investment in the NHS will have increased considerably by the year 2007–08. In return for this, the NHS will offer the following improvements.

- Patients will be admitted for treatment within a maximum of 18 weeks from referral by their GP, and those with urgent conditions will be treated much faster than this.

- Patients will be able to choose between a range of providers, including NHS foundation trusts and treatment centres.

- Patients will be able to be treated at any facility that meets NHS standards, within the national maximum price that the NHS pays for the treatment that they need.

- Patients will have access to a wider range of service in primary care, including access to services nearer their workplace.

- Electronic prescribing will improve the efficiency and quality of prescribing.

- Users of social care will be empowered by the expansion of direct payments.

- In every care setting the quality of care will continue to improve.

- Patients with complex long-term conditions will be supported locally by a new type of clinical specialist, known as a community matron.

Major investment in services closer to home will ensure that there is much better support for patients who have long-term conditions, thereby minimising the impact of these conditions on their lives.

Choose and Book policy

Under the Choose and Book policy, from December 2005 the millions of patients who need elective treatment each year will be offered a choice of appointment at one of four or five different locations. These may be NHS trusts, foundation trusts, treatment centres, private hospitals or practitioners with a special interest operating in primary care.

Patients will be able to choose when they go for their treatment, using national electronic booking systems (see Chapter 10 on information technology). Detailed information (e.g. on waiting times for hospitals and clinics) will be available from the NHS website. Appointments will be made at the GP surgery by calling a contact centre online (and eventually via digital television). The Choose and Book policy is being introduced in stages across the country.

All patients who have to wait longer than six months for an operation are already offered a choice of an alternative place of treatment. The NHS Improvement Plan has set a target maximum waiting time of 18 weeks between referral and first outpatient appointment by December 2008. Patients will have the right to choose from any provider that meets the Healthcare Commission's standards within the price that the NHS will pay.

Quality

The principle is that every part of the NHS and everyone who works in this organisation should take responsibility for working to improve quality. This has to be quality in its broadest sense – that is, doing the right things at the right time for the right people, and doing them right first time. It must cover the quality of the patient's experience as well as the clinical outcomes – that is, quality measured in terms of prompt access, good relationships and efficient administration. This is achieved by means of the programmes, frameworks, authorities and agencies described below.

National Service Frameworks

National Service Frameworks (NSFs) are evidence-based programmes that set out quality standards and state those services that should be available for a specific health condition or care group throughout the health service. NSFs should prevent local variations in the availability of services and standards, and should raise standards and help to improve the health of the nation.

The Department of Health manages the overall process and supports the groups of healthcare professionals, patients, carers and others involved in the development of NSFs.

The programme of NSFs commenced in 1998 and covers the following conditions and care groups:

- mental health (1999)

- coronary heart disease (2000)

- cancer (2000)

- older people (2001)

- diabetes (2001, 2003)

- renal services (part one, 2004, part two, 2005)

- children, young people and maternity services (2004)

- long-term conditions (2005).

A standards-driven system

In April 2005 a new performance framework for the NHS, driven by *Standards for Better Health*, was introduced, which sets out the level of quality that all organisations providing NHS care will be expected to meet or aspire to across the NHS in England.

Standards for Better Health represents the Government's response to a consultation on healthcare standards which was launched in February 2004, and puts quality at the forefront of the agenda both for the NHS and for private and voluntary sector providers of care. The standards describe the level of quality that healthcare organisations, including NHS foundation trusts and private and voluntary sector providers of NHS care, will be expected to meet in terms of safety, clinical and cost-effectiveness, governance, patient focus, accessible and responsive care, care environment and amenities, and public health. A new performance framework for the NHS and social care came into effect in April 2005, setting out the level of quality to be met for all organisations (as noted above) that provide healthcare based on these standards.

Standards for Better Health will form a key part of the performance assessment by the Healthcare Commission (HC) of all healthcare organisations to ensure that the health services provided are both safe and of an acceptable quality.

Clinical governance

Clinical governance is the framework that makes all NHS staff accountable for quality improvement and ensuring that standards and quality remain a priority. Clinical governance has been defined by the Chief Medical Officer as follows:

> a system through which NHS organisations are accountable for continuously improving the quality of their services and safeguarding high standards of care, by creating an environment in which clinical excellence will flourish. It seeks to transform the culture, ways of working and systems of every health organisation so that patient safety, quality assurance and improvement are an integral part of their everyday work. Its main features are a coherent approach to

quality improvement, clear lines of accountability for clinical quality systems, and effective processes for identifying and managing risk and addressing poor performance.

Clinical governance is a new statutory duty, which is intended to ensure that all patients receive quality healthcare. Doctors and other healthcare professionals in both primary and secondary care will take on a legal responsibility for standards of health service treatment.

Clinical governance brings together financial controls and good practice to improve performance. Quality will become an issue for everyone working in the NHS, both in clinical care and in management.

The main principles of clinical governance are as follows:

- an ability to identify easily where both responsibility and accountability lie for the overall quality of medical care, wherever they are provided

- the use of a well-planned package of tools designed to improve the quality of health services, including clinical audit (which evaluates the results of treatment) and medical practice (which is based on research evidence and putting into place medical standards and guidelines)

- providing good staff education and training plans

- clear internal policies aimed at reducing the risk involved with any health service or medical treatment

- clear guidelines for self-regulation which can be applied to all professional groups in order to identify and remedy poor performance.

Primary care groups and trusts, and NHS trusts are accountable for clinical governance and must ensure the quality of their health service and medical treatment.

Healthcare Commission

The Healthcare Commission is independent of the Government, and reports to Parliament. Its main duties are as follows:

- assessing the management, provision and quality of NHS healthcare, including public health

- reviewing every trust's performance and awarding an annual performance rating

- publishing information about the state of healthcare

- considering complaints about NHS organisations that cannot be resolved locally

- promoting the co-ordination of reviews and assessments conducted by others

- regulating the independent healthcare sector through registration, annual inspection and enforcement

- investigating serious failures in the provision of healthcare.

It co-ordinates the activity of other bodies involved in inspecting health-care, and has agreed a concordat aimed at reducing the burden of inspection on frontline healthcare staff, thus playing an important part in quality and audit. This commits each inspectorate to minimising disruption and duplication, ensuring that information is shared and encouraging joint inspections.

The Healthcare Commission will merge with the Commission for Social Care Inspection by 2008. Once the legislation has been passed, the Commission will take over the function of the Mental Health Act Commission.

Quality of services and audit

An important NHS goal is to improve the quality of services to individual patients, their carers and the wider community. One concern of the NHS is to ensure that both the quality and standard of healthcare are consistent across the UK. In your own organisation you may be part of a team involved in customer-care training or developing an improved patient complaints procedure. You have the privilege of being the patient's first point of contact with the clinical team, and you are in an ideal position to identify the non-clinical needs of the patient.

Audit

Clinical audit is the systematic and critical analysis of the quality of clinical care, including the procedures used for diagnosis, treatment and care, the associated resources, and the resulting outcome and quality of life for the patient (Policy Statement on the Development of Clinical Audit).

Clinical audit embraces the audit activity of all healthcare professionals, including doctors, nurses and other healthcare staff. Audit should:

- be professionally led

- be seen as part of an educational process

- form part of routine clinical care

- be based on setting standards

- yield results that help to improve the outcome of the quality of care

- involve management in the process and outcomes of audit
- be confidential at the individual patient or clinical level
- take into consideration the views of the patient and their carer
- be an important part of quality programmes.

The role of receptionists and secretaries in quality and audit

Secretaries and receptionists play an important part in the process of patient care, through their administrative work and their contact with patients. They are often asked to participate in audit activity, for example:

- by recording the time at which each patient arrives at the surgery or clinic, and the actual time when they are seen by a doctor
- by attendance at audit meetings to discuss ways of improving standards.

Remember that the patient's viewpoint and opinion play an important part in audit, and that both secretaries and receptionists are in a good position to hear this view expressed.

Patient and Public Involvement Forums

Patient and Public Involvement Forums (PPIFs) currently exist for every NHS trust and primary care trust, but they will be reconfigured so that one PPIF represents each primary care trust area. Their roles are as follows:

- to monitor and review NHS delivery
- to seek the views of the public about those services
- to make recommendations to the NHS based on this information.

Anyone can apply to be a PPIF member, and currently there are approximately 5000 members.

DH Director for Patients and the Public

In 2003, the DH created the post of National Director for Patients and the Public. The director's role can be summarised as follows:

- to champion the voice of patients, carers and the public throughout the NHS and the DH

- to support staff in working in partnership with the above, and to be responsive to their needs

- to act as a national spokesperson in promoting and explaining patient-focused policy.

The Director reports to the Chief Nursing Officer, who has board-level responsibility for the DH's targets to improve patient experience of the NHS.

National Institute for Clinical Excellence

The National Institute for Clinical Excellence (NICE) is a special authority that was set up in April 1999 to provide guidance for healthcare professionals, managers, patients and carers in making decisions about treatment and healthcare. This covers the following:

- technology appraisals

- clinical guidelines

- the use of new surgical (or other interventional) procedures.

It gives advice on best clinical practice in the NHS to those commissioning NHS services (health authorities and primary care trusts), and to patients and their carers. NICE is a partnership between the Department of Health, the NHS, health professionals and patients. Guidelines set by NICE will be used across the country, helping to end the geographical variations in care that have developed in recent years.

Further information can be found at www.nice.org

National Patient Safety Agency

The National Patient Safety Agency (NPSA) has taken over from the national body, namely the National Clinical Assessment Agency, set up in 2001. It aims to harness systematic learning from patient safety incidents and service failure in the NHS, collecting and analysing information from local NHS organisations, staff, patients and carers, and initiating preventive measures that the whole service can learn from each case. It ensures that where risks are identified, work is undertaken to find solutions, and it specifies national goals and mechanisms to track progress.

The NPSA aims to promote an open and fair culture across the health service, encouraging staff to report incidents and near misses.

The NPSA has taken over responsibility from NICE for three organisations that undertake research into the way in which patients are treated. These National Confidential Enquiries cover suicide and homicide, child and maternal health, and patient outcome and death. The NPSA also leads nationally on hospital food and aspects of hospital design, as well as providing a clinical assessment service to support employers who are concerned about the performance of an individual doctor.

A new key organisation: NHS Institute for Learning, Skills and Innovation

This is a new special health authority that was set up in 2005. It will integrate, promote and support innovation, learning, leadership and improvement. It replaces the NHS University, the NHS Modernisation Agency and the NHS Leadership Centre.

The institute's role will be to help to develop, disseminate and commercialise innovative work in the NHS and the healthcare industry.

Health Action Zones

Health Action Zones (HAZs) are partnerships between the NHS, local authorities, the voluntary and private sectors and local communities. They were introduced by the Department of Health in 1998, and aimed to develop new ways of tackling health inequalities in England's most deprived areas.

Health Development Agency (HDA)

The HDA is a special health authority that aims to improve the health of people in England, and in particular to reduce inequalities in health between those who are well off and those who are on low incomes or reliant on state benefits. The HDA came into force in April 2000. The establishment of the HDA was announced in the White Paper *Saving Lives: our healthier nation*, in the summer of 1999. The White Paper aims to improve the health of everyone, particularly those who are worst off, taking into account the social, economic and environmental factors that affect health. The HDA's role in achieving this aim is to:

- gather evidence of what works

- advise on good practice

- support all those who are working to improve the public's health.

The remit of the HDA is health improvement – involving not just the NHS but also national and local government, and the voluntary, academic and private sectors – to support informed decision making and to develop effective practice.

Health Promotion in England (HPE)

HPE was established in April 2000 following the closure of the Health Education Authority. It develops and delivers public education campaigns and promotes healthy living by focusing in particular on the following:

- alcohol
- children and families
- drugs
- immunisation
- older people
- sexual health.

It works in partnership with national and local organisations (both statutory and voluntary), to provide support to health and other professionals at local and community level. It is part of the NHS and works under contract to the Department of Health and the Department of Trade and Industry.

Resource allocation in the NHS

The Treasury is responsible for overall public expenditure. Every two years it conducts a spending review of all Government departments. The Department of Health, which is also a public department, draws up a public service agreement with the Treasury setting out what it is expected to provide with its new resources over a three-year period. The Department of Health in turn also issues information about priorities and planning guidance to the NHS.

Spending on the NHS is divided into the following programmes.

- *Hospital and community health services, and discretionary family health services*. This covers hospital and community health services, prescribing costs for drugs and appliances, and discretionary General Medical Services (which include reimbursements of General Medical Services, GPs' practice staff, premises, out-of-hours and information technology expenses). It also covers other centrally funded initiatives (e.g. education and training, and research and development).

- *Non-discretionary family health services*. This covers demand-led family health services, including the remuneration of GPs (e.g. capitation payments, health promotion and basic practice allowance), the cost of general dental and ophthalmic services, dispensing remuneration and income from dental and prescription charges.

- *Central health and miscellaneous services*. This includes, for example, some public health functions and support to the voluntary sector.

- *Administration of the Department of Health*.

Primary care trusts

Since 2003–04 the DH has made allocations covering a three-year period direct to PCTs, which now control approximately 80% of the NHS budget. They have to plan their use of resources over the three years as agreed with their strategic health authority.

These unified budget allocations cover the following:

- commissioning hospital, mental health and learning disability services

- providing community services

- PCT running costs

- GPs' and community nurses' prescribing costs

- primary care infrastructure.

Provided that they achieve their targets and keep sufficient in reserve to pay GPs, PCTs can use their resources as they see fit.

PCTs draw up service agreements with healthcare providers to commission services, mostly NHS trusts.

NHS trusts derive most of their income from providing services, although some income is derived from the provision of private healthcare. They are funded separately for training healthcare professionals. They may also generate income from shops and/or car parks on hospital premises.

NHS trusts and PCTs have to publish their costs for individual procedures. These give details of the unit costs for a range of treatments, ranging from X-rays to transplant surgery, and from a visit by a district nurse to a home delivery by a midwife.

Weighted capitation

A weighted-capitation formula is used to determine each PCT's target share of resources. This reflects the age distribution of the PCT's population and the specific health needs it may have due to deprivation or high mortality and morbidity levels, as well as unavoidable geographical variations in the cost of providing services. It is intended that every PCT should be able to commission similar levels of health services for populations with similar need. A wide-ranging review of the formula to make it fairer and to reduce the number of health inequalities was recently conducted by the Advisory Committee on Resource Allocation. The formula takes into account the following:

- hospital and community health services

- HIV/AIDS

- GP practice infrastructure (e.g. practice staff wages, premises and equipment)

- GP prescribing costs (drug costs of prescriptions dispensed, not dispensing fees)

- GP remuneration.

These components are used to adjust each PCT's 'crude population' (based on 2001 census estimates). Some will currently be funded above their target level and others will be funded below it (distance from target), reflecting the legacy of previous years' allocations. Ministers decide each allocation on the basis of the level of increase that all PCTs receive in order to deliver on local and national priorities and the level of extra resources to PCTs that are under target, to move them closer to their weighted-capitation targets.

Payment by results

A system of payment by results is being introduced in an attempt to ensure that funding follows the patient. This is designed to underpin Government policy on increasing patient choice and encouraging a diversity of providers. The changes are being implemented gradually over five years up to 2008 in order to monitor the effect and reduce the risks of financial destabilisation.

The aim is to provide a system for paying trusts which will encourage a reduction in waiting times. PCTs will commission the volume of activity required for their populations, but instead of drawing up block agreements with NHS trusts as previously, the trusts and other providers will be paid for the activity that they undertake. They will lose money on a cost-per-case basis for failing to deliver the volumes commissioned, and will earn extra on a cost-per-case basis for treating additional patients.

A tariff derived from national reference costs will remove prices from local negotiations, so that commissioners focus instead on gains in patient choice, quality, shorter waiting time, volumes of activity and efficiency. Initially the tariff was applied to 15 healthcare resource groups (HRGs) for elective procedures in ophthalmology, cardiothoracic surgery, ENT, trauma and orthopaedics, general surgery and urology.

HRGs classify patients into clinically similar groups that require similar levels of resources for diagnosis, treatment and care. The NHS

Information Authority has developed HRGs in collaboration with clinicians to reflect clinical practice and patterns of delivery.

A further 33 HRGs have recently been added, and from now until 2008 the system will extend to cover most significant inpatient, day-case and outpatient activity.

This reformation of financial flow is one of the most significant changes in which the NHS operates.

The New NHS: modern, dependable

The Labour Government's first health White Paper, published in December 1997, shortly after they came into power, announced the setting up of primary care groups (forerunners of PCTs), NICE and NHS Direct, and described a new model for a new century, based on the following six principles:

- renewing the NHS as a genuinely national service, offering fair access to consistently high-quality, prompt and accessible services across the country

- making delivery of healthcare a social responsibility, with local doctors and nurses shaping services

- getting the NHS to work in partnership, breaking organisational barriers and forging stronger links with local authorities

- driving efficiency through a more rigorous approach to performance

- shifting the focus on to quality of care in order to guarantee excellence for all patients, with quality being the driving force for decision making at every level

- rebuilding public confidence in the NHS as a public service that is accountable to patients, open to the public and shaped by their views.

Delivering care

Primary care

Primary care is the setting in which 90% of NHS patients receive treatment. Due to recent advances in diagnostics and minor surgery, many treatments and procedures that were once carried out in hospital can now be performed in primary care. This trend is more convenient to patients, and reduces the workload for secondary care, especially as many patients are now able to see their GP within two working days, or a primary care professional within one working day, as recommended by the Department of Health guidelines.

Supersurgeries

The NHS Plan described the GP surgery of the future as follows:

> Many GPs will be working in teams from modern multi-purpose premises alongside nurses, pharmacists, dentists, therapists, opticians, midwives and social care staff. Nurses will have new opportunities, and some GPs will tend to specialise in treating different conditions. The consulting room will become the place where appointments for outpatients and operations are booked, test results are received and more diagnosis is carried out using video and tele-links to hospital specialists. An increasing number of consultants will take outpatient sessions in local primary care centres.

PCTs are considering setting up new 'one-stop' health centres which would bring together GPs, health visitors, dentists and optometry services. Work on a number of these centres is under way at the time of writing.

Practitioners with a special interest

GPs with a special interest (GPSIs) have the necessary expertise to provide a specialised clinical service or undertake advanced procedures. They are able to take referrals from colleagues for some conditions/specialties (e.g. dermatology, ophthalmology and ear, nose and throat conditions) and in some instances they are able to undertake minor surgical procedures or to perform diagnostic procedures such as endoscopy. They do not replace consultants in any way.

GPSIs help to reduce patient waiting times and provide a convenient service for many patients, and they also help to free up consultant time in secondary care services.

Walk-in centres

Walk-in centres provide quick access to advice and treatment for minor problems without the need to make an appointment. They are open seven days a week from early morning until the evening, and provide the following services:

- assessment by an experienced NHS nurse
- treatment for minor injuries and illnesses
- instant access to health advice and information on other local out-of-hours GP and dental services
- information on pharmacy services.

Walk-in centres opened in 2000, and an expansion programme is under way. A few instant-access GP centres have been opened which provide physiotherapy, treatment for minor injuries and prescriptions. They are usually close to mainline or underground stations, so are easily accessible for commuters.

As walk-in centres develop further, it is proposed that they will offer independent prescribing by nurses and access to GP services, thus enabling more patients to receive treatment without having to go to their own practice.

NHS Direct

NHS Direct opened in March 1998 and offers fast and free 24-hour advice on personal healthcare. NHS Direct nurses aim to provide callers with the advice and reassurance which they need to care for themselves at home – or if they require further help, to direct them quickly to the right service at the right time. If a condition is more serious or if it is an emergency, nurses can give quick advice on what action the caller should take and, if appropriate, will call an ambulance. Information and advice about the most common illnesses and a range of treatments is now also available on NHS Direct online (www.nhsdirect.nhs.uk).

NHS Direct also provides information about local healthcare services, such as doctors, dentists and late-night pharmacies.

NHS Direct Online (www.nhsdirect.nhs.uk)

This is an interactive website that provides the following information:

- a self-help guide to treating common ailments at home
- a health encyclopaedia
- a 'body key' for identifying symptoms
- a response to requests for information
- a database of community health services, hospitals, GPs, dentists, pharmacies and opticians.

NHS Direct Online provides free access to advice and information. Information points are found in public places such as hospitals, libraries, pharmacies and supermarkets.

NHS Direct Interactive

NHS Direct Interactive is a health information service that is being developed for the interactive area on digital television. It has around 3000 pages of content, including a health encyclopaedia, health topics, a directory of local NHS services and information about using the NHS. It was launched on Sky digital TV in 2004, and will also become available on other digital TV programmes (Freeview and cable).

Other primary care services

These include the following:

- dental services
- pharmaceutical services
- ophthalmic services.

These primary healthcare services will be covered in more detail in Chapter 12.

Dental services

In recent years, NHS dental services have decreased, with many patients finding it virtually impossible to visit an NHS dentist. It is intended that in the near future the budget for primary dental services will be devolved to PCTs so that they can commission primary dental care. This budget will cover surgery salaries and expenses, and dental surgeries will be encouraged to increase their range of services. Please see Chapter 12 for more detailed information.

Community pharmacies

The new pharmacy contract (published in 2005) aims to improve the range and quality of services offered by community services and to integrate these services further into the NHS. The new contract includes three tiers of service.

1 *Essential services* must be provided by all community pharmacists. They include dispensing, disposal of medication and support with regard to self-care.

2 *Advanced services* require that premises meet certain standards and that pharmacists have accreditation. This includes medicines use, review and prescription intervention.

3 *Enhanced services* are commissioned locally by PCTs. These services include minor ailment schemes and smoking cessation services.

Opticians

There are three types of registered opticians.

1   *Optometrists or ophthalmic opticians* carry out eye tests, look for signs of disease, and prescribe and fit glasses and contact lenses. They are graduates who are registered with the General Optical Council. Optometrists are independent contractors, and some of them have specialist skills (e.g. paediatrics, contact lenses or low vision).

2   *Dispensing opticians* fit and sell glasses. They interpret prescriptions but they do not test eyes. Some dispensing opticians sell low-vision aids, and some are qualified to fit contact lenses under supervision by an optometrist.

3   *Ophthalmic medical practitioners* are doctors who specialise in eyes and eye care. They are also independent contractors.

Ophthalmologists are doctors who specialise in eye diseases and perform eye surgery. They usually work in hospital eye departments.

Orthoptists treat disorders of binocular vision and work in eye departments under the supervision of ophthalmologists. They may also carry out visual screening of children in the community.

Under a system of shared care, optometrists may undertake certain clinical procedures, working to an agreed protocol. These may include conditions such as diabetes, cataracts, glaucoma and minor eye problems, and are designed to relieve hospitals and GPs as well as to move patient care into the community. Optometrists are currently pressing for independent and supplementary prescribing rights.

PCTs are responsible for managing optometrists' contracts.

Intermediate care

The intermediate tier of care is an important part of the programme to improve the health and well-being of older people and to improve the quality of services that they receive. This tier of care aids faster recovery from illness, supports timely discharge from hospital and maximises the ability of older people to live independently. These services include the following:

* hospital-at-home schemes

* supported-discharge teams

* nurse-led facilities in acute or community settings

* council-run or independent residential rehabilitation.

Intermediate care includes both health and social care, as well as housing, and relies on partnerships between organisations and professions. It is the key to caring for long-term conditions in the community (*see also* Chapter 12).

Secondary care

Hospitals

Acute hospitals have always been at the forefront of secondary healthcare, and have dominated spending and provision. The Government has pledged that it will expand the NHS's capacity in order to improve access to services and offer patients choice. This means that in addition to the traditional hospital-based secondary care, alternative means of accessing care will be introduced.

The smaller district general hospitals have difficulty in recruiting staff, and are experiencing retention problems.

Medical, scientific and technological advances have made it possible to undertake more procedures as day cases or in primary care settings, gradually blurring the boundaries between the acute sector and the community.

Treatment centres

Treatment centres are units that perform planned surgery and provide treatment in areas that have traditionally had the longest waiting times. As they are separate from unplanned care/treatment, the risk of cancellation of procedures is greatly reduced.

Treatment centres are developing new staff roles, such as perioperative specialist practitioners, advanced nurse practitioners/advisers, and healthcare assistant technicians in radiology, ophthalmology and surgery.

The essential features of a treatment centre include the following:

• delivering a high volume of routine treatments and/or diagnostics as a streamlined service using defined pathways

• planned and booked services, with the emphasis on patient choice or convenience.

Treatment centres are being developed on various models. For example, some will be run by the NHS, by the independent sector or by overseas providers, while others will be funded by public–private partnerships. They may be:

• *virtual treatment centres* – defined services within existing hospitals, using care pathways to ensure efficiency and optimise the patient's experience

• *stand-alone new-build treatment centres* – purpose built and designed for maximum efficiency

• *refurbished sites* – giving fast and easy access to suitable buildings.

Their work falls into three categories:

1   short-stay inpatient work, often in only one capacity (e.g. ortho-
    paedics, ophthalmology)

2   day-case or outpatient work (referred to as 'surgi-centres')

3   community-based diagnostic centres (e.g. endoscopy, ultrasound, and
    minor surgical procedures such as vasectomies and excision of cysts
    and lesions).

Although NHS treatment centres enable the NHS to treat patients more
quickly, there is a possibility that the future of some hospitals may be
threatened because of the removal of large amounts of their work. Therefore the location and specialty of treatment centres must be carefully
decided.

NHS Elect aims to provide support to NHS treatment centres to help
them to improve both clinical quality and patient experience and offer a
consistently high standard of care.

Ambulance and emergency service

The ambulance and emergency service is undergoing major changes,
driven by a ten-year strategy, *Reforming Emergency Care*. Faster ambulance times and better training and equipment for ambulance crews are
considered to be of prime importance. The DH is considering issues such
as how the ambulance and emergency service can be better integrated
with other parts of the NHS, and education and training needs.

The ambulance service responds to 999 calls, urgent admission
requests, high-dependency and inter-hospital transfers, referrals from
NHS Direct and major incidents. In many areas the ambulance trust also
provides transport to hospitals for patients with appointments or who
require other non-emergency treatment.

Emergency calls are prioritised into three categories:

•   category A – immediately life-threatening

•   category B – serious

•   category C – non-serious injury or illness.

Many ambulances use satellite navigation systems, and it is expected that
in the near future all emergency vehicles will carry equipment such as
ECG machines, and will also be equipped with telemetry, which enables
crews to send information about a patient's condition directly to the
receiving hospital.

It has recently been announced that the number of ambulance trusts will be cut from 31 to around 15, after a service review identified a widespread need for high-calibre senior managers.

The national ambulance review, *Taking Healthcare to the Patient: transforming the NHS ambulance services*, sets new rules on how response times should be recorded.

The number of traditional fully equipped ambulances is likely to be reduced over the next few years as the number of vehicles staffed by highly trained emergency care practitioners increases. Ambulance services will take on more diagnostic roles in people's homes, particularly for those whose condition or transport situation make it difficult for them to access hospital.

Mental health services

Mental health is one of the Government's core national priorities, with new services and higher staffing levels being introduced. It would appear that approximately one in four people seeks treatment and help for a mental health problem at some time in their life. Depression alone is costing as much to treat as coronary heart disease.

Mental health services are provided as part of both primary and secondary care, and responsibility is divided between the NHS, social services and voluntary services. PCTs are responsible for commissioning mental health services. There are also 74 specialist mental health trusts which provide the following:

- acute inpatient care

- community and rehabilitation services

- residential care centres

- day hospitals

- drop-in centres.

Many mental health trusts are integrated with social care and are called 'partnership trusts'.

Primary and community services

The majority of patients with mental health disorders, including serious mental health problems, use only primary care services. Despite this, most of the NHS funding for mental health services is spent on inpatient services. Very few professionals (GPs and nurses) in GP surgeries have mental health training, so the more complex cases are referred to the local mental health trust. These patients are then cared for by a consultant psychiatrist-led community mental health team (CMHT). CMHTs include community psychiatric nurses, psychologists, doctors, social workers and occupational therapists.

Mental health services in the community include the following:

- prompt intervention by teams which aim to treat mental illness as soon and as effectively as possible

- assertive outreach teams to provide intensive support for severely mentally ill people

- a home treatment and crisis response to provide flexible acute care in patients' own homes. A 24-hour service is available if required.

Inpatient services

Many of the services that were once provided in hospitals are now provided in the community, and as a result the number of psychiatric inpatient beds has been considerably reduced over the years. However, there is currently a rising demand for inpatient mental care which has increased the pressure on hospital services, with psychiatric beds experiencing high occupancy rates. Acute inpatient services mainly cater for patients detained under the Mental Health Act who are suffering from severe mental illness.

Forensic mental health services

Forensic mental health services provide care for patients with severe mental disorder requiring physical security, who have demonstrated challenging behaviour that is beyond the scope of general psychiatric services. Some of these patients may be mentally disordered offenders. The services that are available fall into three categories:

1 *low-secure units* – locked wards often based near general psychiatric wards in NHS hospitals

2 *medium-secure units* – which operate on a regional basis, consist of locked wards and have a greater number and wider range of staff

3 *high-secure services* – provided by three special hospitals (Ashworth, Broadmoor and Rampton), which offer a higher level of security and care for patients who are potentially a serious risk to others.

The trend is for many patients to be transferred from high-secure units into medium-secure units nearer their homes, designed to provide a more suitable environment.

More services are being developed in the community to provide for the needs of mentally disordered offenders in the community.

The National Service Framework for Mental Health (published in 1999) sets out a ten-year programme to introduce new standards of care that people will be entitled to expect in every part of the country. It includes, for example, mental health promotion (and aims to reduce discrimination and social exclusion), primary care and access to services, effective services for people with severe mental illness (ensuring consistent help for people with mental health needs), caring about carers, and suicide prevention.

In a five-year assessment, the national director for mental health has indicated a need to focus on whole-community mental health.

Public health

Public health is concerned with improving the population's health, rather than with treating the diseases of individual patients. The official definition of public health, devised by a former Chief Medical Officer, is 'the science and art of preventing disease, prolonging life and promoting health through the organised efforts of society'. This aim can only be achieved through partnerships across Government departments and between the Government, the NHS, local authorities and the private and public sectors.

The Government's White Paper *Choosing Health* (published in 2004) is based on the principle that the NHS aims to prevent disease and improve health, not merely to provide treatment for those who are ill. The Secretary of State for Health has been quoted as saying that 'Now is the right time to refocus the NHS to tackle the causes of ill-health and reduce inequalities'.

The Government's view is that people should make their own choices about their lifestyle, and consequently their health, but that their decision making should be supported by good information and advice about the choices available.

The measures covered in the White Paper include the following:

- a ban on smoking in the workplace – restaurants that serve alcohol and pubs that prepare food must ban smoking unless they apply for a special licence
- an overhaul of sexual health services
- action to safeguard children's health (e.g. tackling unhealthy food promotion)
- a specialist obesity service in every PCT.

The public health workforce consists of people who work in one of three categories:

1 health improvement and reducing inequalities – teachers, social workers, local government staff and voluntary sector workers, as well as healthcare professionals

2 public health practice, environmental health officers, health visitors and those who have public health science or health promotion skills in specific fields

3 public health consultants and specialists.

Reducing health inequalities

Unemployment and poor housing are major causes of ill health, and the Government is taking action to tackle health inequalities and thus improve health. The programme for action involves a range of local, regional and national organisations, including the NHS, local authorities, social services, education, planning and employment. Figure 1.4 illustrates the programme for tackling health inequalities.

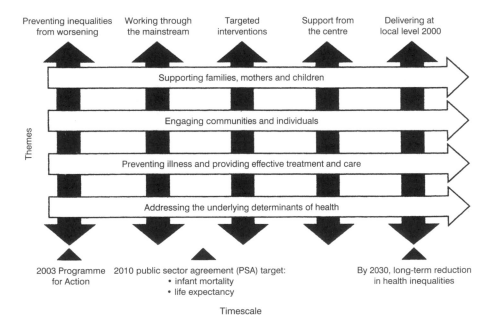

Figure 1.4 Tackling health inequalities: programme for action (Department of Health, 2003).

Public health observatories

Public health observatories are closely linked to the regional public health groups. Their role is to support local bodies by:

* monitoring trends in health and disease issues, and highlighting areas for action

* identifying gaps in health information

* advising on methods for assessing the impact of health inequalities

* drawing together information from different sources in new ways in order to improve health

* carrying out projects to highlight particular health issues

* evaluating progress by local agencies in improving health and reducing inequality

* looking ahead to give early warning of public health problems.

Further information can be found at www.pho.org.uk

Healthy Living Centres (HLCs)

Healthy Living Centres are an initiative managed by the New Opportunities Fund, launched in 1999, and have a budget from Lottery funds to develop a network of HLCs.

This programme targets the most disadvantaged areas and groups in society. HLCs are expected to influence social exclusion, poor access to services and the social and economic inequalities of deprivation.

Projects include smoking cessation services, dietary advice, promotion of physical activity, health screening programmes, training and skills schemes, and complementary therapy.

The NHS, the regions and devolution

The Bevan concept of a 'national' health service in the 1940s went the way of all good ideas with the advent of devolution. Devolution has meant the inception of the Welsh Assembly, the Northern Ireland Assembly and the Scottish Parliament. The different countries of the UK are now taking care of their own business. In other words, there are four national health services.

Somehow we are to be persuaded that healthcare in Scotland, Wales and Northern Ireland is so different from healthcare in England that it has to be run separately, funded separately, employ people separately and be planned for separately. On the one hand, you might argue that local people making local decisions about local priorities is no bad thing. On the other hand, there is never-ending duplication as largely English initiatives are copied in Scotland, Wales and Northern Ireland, and duplication of institutions and planning does not come cheap.

The NHS in Scotland

The whole of Scotland is only the size of an English region. However, the geography is very challenging. Health services have to be provided for communities as diverse as the Orkney Islands and the tenements of Glasgow.

The Scottish Executive Health Department (SEHD) oversees the work of the Scottish NHS. It reports to the Scottish Health Minister, who is an elected member of the Scottish Parliament.

Funding for all services in Scotland is allocated by the British Chancellor in the Westminster budget. The allocation of funds for the Scottish NHS is then decided upon by Scottish ministers, usually on a 'what it was last year and a bit for inflation' principle. Once the health funding figure is known, the Scottish Finance Minister and the Scottish Parliament divide the global sum as they see fit.

There are 15 NHS boards in Scotland (12 boards on the mainland and three island boards). Their roles are organisation, accountability and governance of the system, and the delivery of Local Health Plans (LHPs).

The next layer of administration was 28 NHS trust hospitals. However, from April 2004, in a reorganisation described in the White Paper *Partnership for Care*, trust status was removed and the hospitals now report directly to the boards, which are now known as Unified Boards.

Hospitals were not the only part of the service to be reorganised. Originally primary care services, family services and community and mental health services were planned and provided by PCTs. They have also been swept aside and have become operating divisions of the Unified Boards. The aim of the reorganisation is to devolve as much of the decision making as possible to frontline staff.

These changes were piloted in the Borders and Dumfries and Galloway areas. There is some flexibility in the system, and other areas may, over time, devolve their own management structures.

Community Health Partnerships (CHPs), which involve groups of GPs with the aim of providing services to patients, developing clinical priorities and supporting LHPs, have replaced the original Local Healthcare Co-operatives. The CHPs work closely with local authorities and report to the Unified Boards. Their overall objective is to improve the health of local communities.

The SEHD manages the whole system through a process of annual review. It publishes an annual list of targets and priorities. Local providers, the hospitals and CHPs are then required to submit their plans for reaching the targets.

If this sounds a bit top-down, the answer is that it is! However, community planning is important. CHPs and local authorities publish an annual joint health improvement plan, tackling health gain by working in partnerships. This approach recognises some of the sociodemographic and epidemiological challenges that Scotland faces and acknowledges that the pathway to improve health cannot be achieved by the NHS alone. Housing and other social issues play a major part.

The NHS in Wales

The National Assembly for Wales is responsible for policy direction and for allocating funds to the NHS, but it cannot raise taxes. However, it can create and amend secondary legislation to determine spending priorities.

The future of the NHS in Wales was reviewed in 2002 in a very businesslike document entitled *Structural Change in the NHS*.

As a result, there are now Local Health Boards (LHBs) in every area, serving their own localities in very similar ways to the English arrangement for PCTs. LHBs provide a local focus for the development and improvement of health services. They achieve this by developing Health Improvement Programmes (HImPs), developing the principles of clinical governance to improve the quality of primary healthcare, and informing and developing the commissioning of hospital and community health services.

LHBs consist of local doctors, nurses and other healthcare professionals, and representatives from the local Council (including elected members), voluntary organisations and the public. In addition, a carer will sit on every Board (this arrangement is unique to Wales).

LHBs are stand-alone organisations save for the fact that they are backed up by six Business Service Centres, which provide combined IT and administrative support functions.

NHS trusts run hospitals and community services. There are 15 NHS trusts, including one pan-Wales ambulance trust. These trusts manage 135 hospitals with around 15 000 beds. Services which are too specialised to be dealt with locally will continue to be organised on an all-Wales basis, being delivered in all parts of Wales.

The NHS is the largest employer in Wales, with 60 000 staff, representing more than 7% of the Welsh workforce. There are around 1900 family doctors, 1000 dentists and 600 opticians.

Welsh NHS trusts and health authorities are required by law to consult their Community Health Council (CHC) if they propose major changes in the pattern or provision of services. There is a CHC in each of the 22 local government areas in Wales, and they take up a wide range of health issues on behalf of the public.

The Health and Social Services Secretary in the National Assembly is the minister responsible to the Welsh Assembly Government, who draws up strategic policies for health and health services and allocates resources, configures the NHS in Wales in a way that is consistent with its broader objectives, holds NHS organisations to account for their performance, and promotes the provision of particular services in Wales.

The NHS in Northern Ireland

Just like the rest of the NHS in the UK, Northern Ireland has its fair share of change fever. Added to this are the general problems concerning political instability and the suspension of the Northern Ireland Assembly. As a result, many of the proposed reforms and changes have had to be shelved.

In a document published in March 1999, *Fit for the Future: a new approach*, the Government set out its proposals for the future of the health and personal social services in Northern Ireland.

It established the Department of Health, Social Services and Public Safety, the responsibilities of which include health and personal social services (which includes policy and legislation for hospitals, family practitioner services, community health and personal social services), public health (which includes responsibility for policy and legislation to promote and protect the health and well-being of the population of Northern Ireland) and public safety (which will encompass responsibility for the policy and legislation for the Fire Authority, food safety and emergency planning).

There is an interesting difference in Northern Ireland. Both healthcare and social care are covered by one government department. Some observers say that this makes a great deal of sense.

However, the Northern Ireland Assembly does not raise health taxes, and relies on the conventional Exchequer Grant system. Social services receives its money from local government. As a result, there is often a mismatch in funding.

The Department is run by a Permanent Secretary responsible to the minister, who is an elected politician, and it currently employs about 850 staff. There are over 41 000 staff in the entire health and social services sector.

A total of 15 Local Health and Social Care Groups, based around GP practices and representing natural communities, enable local GPs and other primary care professionals to work in partnership with boards, trusts and the local community with the aim of improving the health and social services for the whole community.

There are six Local Health and Social Care Groups in the Eastern Board area, four in the Northern Board area, three in the Southern Board area and two in the Western Board area. There is huge variation in the populations that they cover. Even taking into account some awkward geography, the populations still range between 60 000 and 200 000.

The so-called Hayes Report, a review of acute hospitals chaired by the former ombudsman Dr Maurice Hayes, which was published in June 2001, proposes radical changes, hospital closures, the building of new hospitals, and changes to the way in which some clinicians are employed. The time scale is 15 years.

Summary

There have been enormous changes in the NHS and medical practice, especially in recent years, and this chapter endeavours to reflect the complexities and the wide range of developments that have taken place since the NHS first came into being in 1948. Everyone working in the field of healthcare, whether in the public or private sector, needs to have an understanding of the changes which are taking place and the policies that are being introduced at the present time.

1988

January	Ministerial Review of the NHS.
July	Department of Health created following the splitting up of the Department of Health and Social Security. Kenneth Clarke appointed as Secretary of State for Health.

1989

January	*Working for Patients* is published.
November	*NHS and Community Care Bill* is published.

1990

June	*NHS and Community Care Bill* receives Royal Assent.

1991

April	NHS reforms come into operation. The first wave of 57 NHS trusts and 306 GP fundholders is established in England.
October	The *Patient's Charter* is published.

1992

April	The second wave of 99 NHS trusts and 288 GP fundholders is established in England.
July	White Paper on *The Health of the Nation* is published.
October	Report of the *Tomlinson Inquiry* is published.

1993

February	The Government publishes its response to the *Tomlinson Inquiry*, entitled *Making London Better*. A review of functions and manpower in the NHS is announced.
April	The third wave of 136 NHS trusts and over 600 GP fundholders is established in England.

July	The functions and manpower review reports to ministers.
October	*Managing the New NHS* is published in response to review. This included the proposed abolition of regional health authorities, the merger of district health authorities and family health services authorities, and a streamlining of the NHS management executive.

1994

April	The fourth wave of 140 NHS trusts and 800 GP fundholders is established in England. The NHS management executive is renamed the NHS Executive and establishes eight regional offices. The number of regional health authorities is reduced from 14 to 8.
June	NHS performances tables published for the first time.
October	*Developing NHS Purchasing and GP Fundholding* is published.

1995

January	An updated *Patient's Charter* is published.
April	The fifth wave of 21 NHS trusts and 560 GP fundholders is established in England. An accountability framework for fundholders is introduced.
June	*Health Authorities Bill* receives Royal Assent.
November	Plans to use a private finance initiative to build a new NHS hospital are announced.

1996

April	Regional health authorities are abolished and their functions are taken over by NHS Executive regional offices. District health authorities and family health services authorities are replaced by unitary health authorities. The sixth wave of 1200 GP fundholders is established in England. Around 50 total purchasing projects go live.
June	Consultation paper, *Primary Care: the future* is published.
October	White Paper on primary care, *Choice and Opportunity*, is published. Reports of NHS funding problems.
November	White Paper on the future of the NHS, *The National Health Service: a service with ambitions*, is published. *The NHS (Primary Care) Bill* is published. Additional resources for the NHS are announced.
December	Second White Paper on primary care, *Primary Care: delivering the future*, is published.

1997

May	A Labour Government is elected and Frank Dobson is appointed Secretary of State for Health.
December	White Paper, *The New NHS: modern, dependable*, is published. White Paper on the future of the NHS in Scotland, *Designed to Care*, is published.

1998
   April   First-wave health action zones (HAZs) established. First wave of newly merged trusts is announced.
1999
   June   *Health Act* received Royal Assent and came into force in April 2000. The new NHS reforms, which included quality of care in NHS trusts and responsibility of partnership between the NHS and local authorities.

   July   Public health White Paper, *Saving Lives: our healthier nation*, is published.
2000
   July   *The NHS Plan – a plan for investment, a plan for reform* is published.

2002   Publication of Wanless Report on healthcare spending needs.
                  New GP and consultant contracts established.

2004   Publication of *NHS Improvement Plan*.
                  Publication of public health White Paper, *Choosing Health*.

References

- Department of Health (2004) *Choosing Health: making healthy choices easier*. Department of Health, London.

- Department of Health (2004) *The NHS Improvement Plan: putting people at the heart of public services*. Department of Health, London.

- Department of Health (2005) *Treatment Centres Delivering Faster Quality Care and Choice for NHS Patients*. Department of Health, London.

- Department of Health (2005) *Supporting People with Long-Term Conditions: an NHS and social model to support local innovation and integration*. Department of Health, London.

Useful websites

www.dh.gov.uk
www.irpanel.org.uk
www.nhselect.org.uk
www.nhsla.com
www.wales.nhs.uk
www.show.scot.nhs.uk
www.n-i.nhs.uk
www.nice.org.uk
www.npps.nhs.uk

2

Patient (customer) care

The medical receptionist and secretary

Medical secretaries and receptionists are important and sometimes undervalued members of the healthcare team. Usually they are the first point of contact that the patient has with a medical practice or a hospital department, clinic or ward. The receptionist's attitude, empathy and efficiency are able either to enhance or to damage their image. A good receptionist can facilitate the way in which a patient accesses the system of medical care, and should do all that is possible to make the patient feel welcome and comfortable, and to ease their access to medical help and care.

The first impression the patient has of the surgery or hospital department is usually of the reception area and the reception staff. Remember that the receptionist is the 'shop window' and the way in which patients feel as they sit in the waiting-area will largely depend on how the receptionist has reacted to and greeted them. It is the receptionist's role to allay patients' fears and worries and help them to feel 'comfortable' whilst they wait. A courteous, friendly manner, accompanied by a smile and an understanding of the situation can work wonders even with the most difficult patients. The secretary, too, often has to reassure anxious patients and their relatives, and should adopt a similar approach.

Everyone, whether they be patients, secretaries, receptionists, doctors or other members of the healthcare team, has feelings. If you have personal problems it is difficult not to let your emotions affect the way in which you respond and interact with patients and colleagues. It is important to be aware of this and develop the ability to overcome your feelings. Your attitude will influence the attitude of the person you are dealing with. Remember that patients have personal problems, too, and are often anxious or frightened, so your empathy with their feelings will do a lot to improve your own attitude.

Box 2.1

How do you welcome patients?

Do you welcome them all in the same way?

Why do you treat people differently?

Why are some patients 'difficult' when they attend a hospital or GP surgery?

What are patients' expectations?

Have you experienced feelings of fear?

How do you react when you are frightened or worried?

How would you like to be treated?

Putting patients first

What is customer care?

Customer care means:

- giving the right impression
- meeting customers' expectations
- exceeding customers' expectations
- listening to customers
- having customer-friendly systems
- being totally professional
- putting customers first
- being totally customer oriented
- having the right attitude
- treating others as you would wish to be treated
- maintaining consistently high standards of service.

Remember that the NHS is a very large business organisation and the customers are your business.

Customer care is **not**:

- a quick fix
- the flavour of the month
- a campaign which runs for three months and then stops
- just something for the receptionists
- something which brings instant results
- something which starts *after* the patient has reported to the receptionist.

What does the customer expect of us?

Customers have a variety of expectations about the following:

- the product and service
- staff
- the organisation – hospital or GP surgery.

These expectations will include the following:

- welcoming, pleasant, smiling receptionists
- a concern for their needs
- interest and recognition
- value for money
- adequate information
- good support services
- satisfaction of their needs
- quality care/service.

Every patient/customer matters and deserves the best that you and your NHS trust, general practice, hospital or clinic can offer.

Creating the right impression

Box 2.2 Some do's and don'ts for creating the right impression

DO	DON'T
Greet the patient pleasantly	Be rude
Make eye contact	Avoid looking at patient
Use patients' or callers' names where known	Be distant, or call everyone 'dear' or 'love'
Give your full attention	Be bored
	Talk to colleagues when patients need attention
Show respect for the patient	Criticise other members of the healthcare team
Be helpful	Be unco-operative
Be confident	
Be positive	
Be efficient	
Be caring	
SMILE	

What improvements can be made?

By you?

By other members of the team?

YOU NEVER GET A SECOND CHANCE TO MAKE
A FIRST IMPRESSION!

A number of factors help to create the right or wrong impression, including the following:

- layout – user-friendly seating
- space

- accessibility

- signs

- noise

- clutter/rubbish

- staff appearance

- staff behaviour

- facial expression

- tone of voice

- posture.

How to discover the customer's needs

Try to pick up any clues from what is said by the customer either in person or on the telephone and listen to the 'hidden' message. Do not jump to conclusions about the customer's needs – they are not always clearly expressed.

Follow up and probe by asking questions. Use 'open' questions, starting with the following.

- How?

- Why?

- What?

- When?

However, do not interrogate the customer.

Actively listen in order to discover the customer's needs

- Do not make hasty judgements.

- Do not let personal feelings or prejudices prevent you from listening to what is being said.

- Do not interrupt, even if you feel that you can guess the end of the sentence or remark.

- Do not forget to show that you are listening.

- Do not be distracted.

Body language or non-verbal communication (NVC)

Body language is an important factor in customer care. Remember that it may reflect what you are really thinking! Body language should reinforce the spoken word. When it is contradictory, the customer may well believe the body language and not what is being said.

Important aspects of body language include the following.

- *Facial expressions and head position* – the face is mobile and can register a huge range of expressions. The expression on your face when you welcome the customer will affect their impression of you. Your head position is also important. Tilting your head to one side indicates interest in the other person.

- *Posture* – the way in which you hold your body is important. Observe people in your place of work and you will be surprised at the information you can obtain from their posture. Posture gives an indication of the level of interest in the customer. For example, leaning slightly towards the customer suggests interest and concern, leaning away with the arms folded indicates lack of interest or even boredom, and standing with the hands on the hips is an aggressive signal.

- *Proximity* – we all need our 'personal space' and people who get too close to us will often make us feel uncomfortable and threatened. You should be close enough to customers to show interest – approximately three to four feet away is usually the best distance.

- *Eye contact and gaze* – looking someone in the eye is generally felt to be a positive signal. Look directly at the customer, albeit briefly, when making the initial welcome. Not looking at them may indicate an attitude of not caring. However, some people avoid eye contact for reasons of shyness or because of cultural tradition. Your eyes probably give the most expressive signal of all. Watch the customer's eyes during a conversation and you will gain feedback as to whether they understand or agree with what you are saying. Aim to meet their gaze for approximately two-thirds of the time.

- *Body contact* – in our society it is not appropriate to touch a complete stranger. In general, the only acceptable form of touching is the handshake when greeting or saying goodbye to a customer.

- *Gestures* – our gestures provide a lot of information (e.g. a nod or a shrug). Negative gestures include finger or foot tapping (impatience or aggression) and yawning (boredom).

- *Tone of voice* – we all convey a great deal of information to people not by what we are saying, but by the tone of our voice. You may use welcoming words, but if you sound uninterested or angry you may cause the patient distress. Always ensure that your tone is as friendly as the actual words spoken.

A good technique is to mirror the customer's body language. Customer care and use of the telephone will be dealt with in Chapter 3.

Complaints within the health service

In recent years there has been increasing public awareness about quality of service. People have higher expectations of the service that they receive. It used to be the case that people only complained if the quality of the goods that they bought was substandard, but nowadays people are equally concerned about how they are treated when they are buying their goods.

This also applies to the health service. People expect to receive a high standard of care and service. If they do not do so, they are becoming more forthright about complaining.

Complaints are taken very seriously in the health service today. In order to develop and maintain a high standard of service, we need to know when things go wrong. We need to know what has happened so that it can be avoided in future, and so that action is taken to prevent it from happening again. Both general practitioners and patients are unlikely to choose a hospital for referral where there is a high level of complaints about which no action is taken.

We also need to respond to our customers, the patients. If they do not receive the service that they expect, they need to know that they can complain and that their complaint will be investigated. They need to know that their complaint will be taken seriously and that they will receive an explanation and apology, if appropriate.

Patients have the right to have any complaints about NHS services investigated, and to receive a full written reply. The following principles have been agreed which should underpin any effective complaints procedure:

- responsiveness
- quality enhancement
- cost-effectiveness
- accessibility
- impartiality
- simplicity
- speed
- confidentiality
- accountability.

These principles provide the foundation for the NHS complaints procedure that was introduced in April 1996. The procedure aims to provide a fair, simple and open system which is easy to access and enables lessons on quality to be extracted and used to improve services for patients. The primary aim is to resolve complaints and satisfy the concerns of the complainant through early, local resolution.

Why do patients complain?

Patients complain about a wide variety of different issues, such as the following:

- postponement of an appointment

- waiting-times for a first outpatient appointment or to see the doctor in the clinic or surgery

- cancellation of an appointment or admission to hospital

- time on the waiting-list

- cancellation or postponement of surgical procedures

- lack of information

- not being kept informed of treatments

- staff behaviour and attitudes

- food

- a doctor not visiting the patient at home

- cleanliness and building debris

- missing medical records, X-rays and test results

- missing property.

The person nominated by the practice or NHS trust to be responsible for dealing with complaints should give information about the procedure to the person who is complaining. This will include, where appropriate:

- how the complaint will be dealt with

- the purpose of the procedure

- the anticipated timetable

- the rules of confidentiality

- the availability of help from the local Patient Advice and Liaison Services (PALS)

- possible outcomes of the procedure, so that the person complaining may have realistic expectations

- the availability of conciliation services through the NHS trusts or health board

- how to pursue a complaint with the health authority or trust if the person who is complaining is not satisfied with the practice-based investigation

- the time limit for making complaints, which is within six months of the event(s) concerned or within six months of becoming aware that there is something to complain about. Primary care practitioners and complaints managers in NHS organisations have discretion to waive this time limit if there are good reasons why the patient or representative could not complain earlier.

Patients have the right to a full and prompt written reply from the Chief Executive to any written complaint against a trust or health authority. The NHS tries to provide this within four weeks of receiving any complaint. Where there are good reasons why this cannot be achieved, patients must be kept informed of progress.

The complaints procedure

The aim of the system is to try to resolve most complaints close to the cause of patients' complaints, be that a doctor, nurse, receptionist, secretary or practice manager. In many cases it should be possible to resolve the problem straight away. This procedure is part of the local resolution mechanism for settling complaints in the NHS.

If patients feel that they have a reason to complain, they can do so directly to the medical practice or NHS organisation concerned. However, health authorities or health boards have complaints managers who may be contacted by patients if they prefer to talk to someone who is not directly involved in their healthcare.

The complaints procedure is currently under review, with no changes expected in the foreseeable future. Inevitably, because of recent changes and mergers in the health service, new procedures will be introduced to reflect these at a future date.

How patients may complain about the NHS

If patients are unhappy with the treatment or service that they received from the NHS, they are entitled to make a complaint, to have it considered and to receive a response from the NHS organisation or primary care practitioner concerned. The following NHS procedure applies to the NHS in England, with the exception of NHS foundation trusts.

A PALS has been established in every NHS trust and primary care trust (PCT). Although PALS are not part of the complaints procedure itself, they may be able to resolve the concerns of patients informally, or to provide more information about the complaints procedure and independent complaints advocacy services.

Local resolution

The NHS complaints procedure covers complaints made by a person about any matter connected with the provision of NHS services by NHS organisations or primary care practitioners (GPs, dentists, opticians and pharmacists). The procedure also covers services provided overseas or by the private sector for which the NHS has paid. Amended Complaints Regulations will be issued once the Department of Health has been able to give proper consideration to any recommendations made by the Shipman Inquiry, which published its fifth report in December 2004.

Who may complain?

A complaint can be made by any patient or person who is affected or likely to be affected by the actions or decisions of an NHS organisation or primary care practitioner. A complaint can also be made by someone acting on behalf of the patient or person, with their consent.

Time limits for making a complaint

Patients (or their representatives) should normally complain within six months of the event(s) concerned, or within six months of becoming aware that there is something to complain about. Primary care practitioners and complaints managers in NHS organisations have discretion to waive this time limit if the patient (or their representative) has good reasons for not complaining earlier. In these circumstances the time limit will be extended from six months to one year.

Procedure

Local resolution

The first stage of the NHS complaints procedure is *local resolution*. In the first instance, complaints should be made to the organisation or primary care practitioner that provided the service. Local resolution aims to resolve complaints quickly and as close to the source of complaint as possible by appropriate means (e.g. conciliation).

Patients or their representatives may raise their concerns by speaking to a member of staff (e.g. GP, dentist, nurse, practice manager) or someone else (e.g. the PALS) who may be able to resolve their concerns, rendering a formal complaint unnecessary. However, if patients or their representatives want to pursue their complaint further, this may be done orally or in writing (including email) to the primary care practitioner or the NHS organisation concerned. If a complaint is made orally, a written record of this should be made by the complaints manager.

The primary care practitioner should reply within ten working days, and the Chief Executive of the NHS organisation concerned should reply within 25 working days. Patients or their representatives should be kept informed of progress if this is not going to happen. A complaint may be made about any matter concerned with NHS services, including decisions that may affect people who are neither current nor former patients. Complaints are often made about access to services.

If a complaint is not resolved within six months, it may be referred to the Healthcare Commission.

NHS organisations and primary care practitioners have a new duty to co-operate in receiving and investigating complaints, and to provide comprehensive responses to complaints.

A board member or other senior person must be designated to ensure that all complaints are considered and investigated, and that action is taken as a result. Complainants must be kept informed at all stages of the process.

Regular reports must be made detailing the numbers of complaints received, the nature of the complaints, and any action taken as a result of the investigation of a complaint.

Private treatment in an NHS hospital

If patients have paid for treatment by a consultant which was provided in an NHS hospital's private section, the NHS complaints procedure will not cover this. Any such complaints should be taken up with the General Medical Council and/or by contacting the consultant directly. However, the NHS procedure will cover any complaint made about the hospital's staff (but not the consultant) or facilities relating to the care provided in its private beds. The complaints manager for the NHS organisation that funded the treatment will give appropriate advice. The independent provider of the treatment should have its own complaints procedure, as required by the Care Standards Act 2000, and this can be used as an alternative to the NHS complaints procedure.

Independent review

In the case of complaints about the NHS and independent health services (including complaints about an NHS foundation trust) which have not been resolved at a local level, the Healthcare Commission may be approached to give an 'independent review'.

NHS foundation trusts

NHS foundation trusts will have their own system for the internal handling of complaints, which may differ from the local resolution process. Patients or their representatives should contact the NHS foundation trust for advice and information on how to make a complaint.

The Ombudsman

The Health Service Ombudsman (Health Service Commissioner) undertakes independent investigations into complaints about the NHS, and will investigate complaints against private healthcare providers only if the treatment was funded by the NHS, although further consideration is not an automatic right. Please refer to Chapter 1 for more detailed information.

Independent Complaints and Advocacy Service (ICAS)

The Independent Complaints and Advocacy Service supports patients and their carers who wish to pursue a complaint about their NHS treatment or care. This statutory service was launched on 1 September 2003, and provides for the first time a national service that is delivered to agreed quality standards.

ICAS empowers clients by providing information, support and guidance to help them to articulate their concerns and navigate the complaints system. This may include assistance with constructing a complaints letter, and drafting plans for or attending meetings.

ICAS supports the principle of local resolution, and aims to help clients to find a solution as close as possible to the point of the service that has caused dissatisfaction, thereby maximising the likelihood of the complaint being resolved quickly and effectively.

ICAS is provided on a regional basis, including the Citizens' Advice Bureaux and the Carer's Federation.

Summary of the NHS complaints procedure

- First stage – local resolution.

- Second stage – independent review.

- Third stage – referral to an Ombudsman.

- Judicial review – it may be possible for the final decision to be challenged by seeking a judicial review. Judicial review procedure allows a court of law to review decisions made by public bodies.

Receptionists and secretaries are advised to ask their managers for a copy of the complaints procedure used in their healthcare organisation, and for any points about which they are unsure to be explained.

Having a standard procedure also ensures clear communication. In fact, lack of communication is the root cause of many of the complaints that are made in hospitals. A complaint about a relatively minor matter can become quite serious if it is not taken seriously in the first place. Thus having a complaints procedure is better both for patients and for staff. It ensures that complaints are taken seriously, and that everyone involved has an opportunity to express their opinion. It encourages clear communication, and by doing so may reduce complaints in the long term. It can also help to improve the hospital's public image. More importantly, the major benefit of having a procedure is to ensure that the quality of service can be monitored, thus helping to maintain and develop high standards of care.

Taking customer complaints seriously

All complaints must be taken seriously. If a customer complains, this provides an opportunity to put things right. All complaints should be:

- logged

- passed to the appropriate manager

- acted upon.

Complaints should be dealt with immediately, and the customer should know the outcome as soon as possible. Remember that a complaint is any situation in which the customer is not satisfied. If a complaint is handled well, the customer might feel more loyalty than before.

Box 2.3 Do's and don'ts of complaints

DO	DON'T
Obtain all of the facts	Interrupt
Listen to what the patient or customer has to say	Argue
	Justify
Apologise on behalf of the organisation without making excuses	Make excuses
	Ignore
Show concern	Forget to explain the procedure
Tell the patient or customer what will be done	

Patients expect:

• an apology, if appropriate

• a clear explanation

• assurance that action will be taken to prevent a recurrence.

Patient and public involvement

To avoid substandard services, patients and the public are involved in the shaping of local services. This was an important aim of the NHS Plan, which wanted to ensure that both patients and the public had a say in how services are planned and developed. The Health and Social Care Act (2001) placed a duty on all NHS organisations and health authorities to 'involve and consult' patients and the public. Under this Act, patients and the public must be involved in the following:

• planning services

• considering proposals for change in the way in which services are provided

• decisions that affect the way in which those services operate.

Patients and the public are now given the opportunity to put forward their ideas for change and to discuss their own experiences and the organisation's plans for future services. They are also invited to suggest what they expect from health services and to give reasons for change, and may be involved in making strategic decisions about how or where services should be provided.

NHS organisations must consider patient and public issues, and must include on the membership of their boards a staff member to be responsible for these issues. Resources must be provided for patient/public involvement, and it must be ensured that all staff receive appropriate training.

The Healthcare Commission is responsible for promoting national patient surveys and using the feedback obtained from these to assess trusts' performance. The NHS Plan requires every trust to obtain feedback from patients about the care that they have received.

Many reforms of patient and public involvement have taken place – for example, abolishing the Community Health Councils which were formed during the 1974 reorganisation, and replacing them with PALS.

Patient and public involvement forums (PPIFs) have been set up in every NHS and PCT. They monitor the operation of their services and also monitor the effectiveness of PALS. They have minimum number of seven members (15–20 being the preferred number). It is proposed that PPIFs should have a member appointed as a non-executive director on the trust board. PPIFs are responsible for the following:

- patients' views about services

- inspecting NHS premises

- making reports and recommendations to trust managers as a result of the experiences of patients and their carers

- monitoring the services on the basis of the patients' expressed views

- referring their concerns to NHS trusts and other organisations as appropriate.

In 2003 the Department of Health created the post of Director for Patients, whose role is to champion the voice of patients, carers and the public in the Department of Health and throughout the NHS, and to support staff to enable them to work in partnership with patients and carers, and to respond to their needs. The director should also act as a national spokesperson in promoting and explaining patient-focused policy.

The director is responsible to the Chief Nursing Officer, who is the director of patient experience of the NHS.

Local councils scrutinise all major changes to local health services. If the council is not satisfied that the planned changes are in the best interests of the local population, it can refer the decision and obtain independent advice and recommendations.

Commission for Patient and Public Involvement in Health (CPPIH)

The CPPIH has been set up to oversee the new system of patient and public involvement, working nationally, regionally and locally to act as a patients' champion. It is an independent, non-departmental public body sponsored by the Department of Health.

The CPPIH sets up, funds and appoints all members to PPIFs, as well as managing their performance. It advises the Secretary of State on how the whole system of patient and public involvement is working, and it reports on these issues to other national bodies. It also conducts national reviews of services from the patient's perspective, collating data from PPIFs and making recommendations.

The CPPIH's head office is in Birmingham and it has nine regional centres across England.

Final impressions

The patient must go away feeling satisfied with the level of service you have given. They should feel that you:

- have been willing to help
- have gone to some trouble
- are more co-operative than others.

This will give a good impression of:

- you
- your communication skills as a secretary or receptionist
- your medical practice, NHS trust, hospital or other healthcare organi-sation.

Don't take customers (i.e. patients) for granted.

Summary

Customer care means that you as a medical secretary or receptionist should ensure:

- that your customers are, and feel, welcome (e.g. the way in which you greet them when they arrive will show them whether you care)

- that you show concern for the customer's needs (e.g. by the way in which you listen when they are asking a question or explaining something)

- that you are interested, friendly and pleasant (e.g. by being courteous at all times)

- that you know what you are talking about (e.g. the services that your hospital, practice or clinic offers)

- that the services are the best possible

- that you recognise each customer as an individual person.

The medical secretary and receptionist and customer care

An experienced receptionist's or secretary's responsibility can be boundless and very fulfilling. They are able to assist and understand patients' medical conditions and help accordingly. They may arrange for a wheelchair, a porter or generally provide assistance. They will notice if a patient appears to be distressed and point this out to a nurse or doctor if they consider it necessary. On a practical level, they will keep the reception area generally tidy. For example, magazines will be up to date and in good condition, toys for children will not become a hazard to waiting patients but are kept in a special play area, and plants and flowers will be fresh and watered when necessary. In a private hospital or practice, coffee will no doubt be offered to patients while they wait.

Patients' rights

Patients' rights with regard to treatment from the family doctor service include the following:

- to be registered with a GP

- to change doctors quickly and easily

- to receive any treatment from a GP which is immediately necessary in an emergency, even if the patient is not registered with them

- to receive treatment outside surgery hours (e.g. from a deputising agency)

- to have appropriate drugs and medicines as prescribed

- to be referred to an acceptable consultant when the family doctor considers this is necessary, and to be referred for a second opinion if the patient and their family consider it desirable

- to have access to personal medical records, subject to any limitations by law

- to know that those working for the NHS are under a legal duty to keep the contents of health records confidential

- to choose whether or not to take part in medical research or student training

- to be given detailed information about local family doctor services

- to receive a copy of the doctor's practice leaflet, setting out the services that they provide

- to receive a full and prompt reply to any complaint made about NHS services.

Access to healthcare

The NHS Plan also commits to improved access to healthcare. Both NHS Direct and NHS walk-in centres provide better access to healthcare.

Consider the ways in which medical secretaries and receptionists ensure that all patients receive the best service and support. This will mean attending to the following:

- the general needs of all patients and visitors

- the special needs of some patients, especially those concerned with mobility, disability, the elderly and ethnic minorities

- patient transport.

Many patients, some of whom will also have special needs, are anxious and uneasy about their visit to the surgery or hospital. The receptionist is usually the first person with whom a patient will communicate, and the special skills, knowledge, understanding and empathy that the receptionist uses when receiving and dealing with the patient are very important.

Patients' general needs

Secretaries and receptionists should be able to answer all queries about the services offered by the practice or hospital department, and to direct patients and give them appropriate information, for example about the following:

- waiting-area

- clinic or surgery times

- relevant consulting-room

- toilet, including disabled facilities

- changing facilities

- refreshment facilities (machines, snack bar, etc.).

Patients' special needs

'Disabled' means being unable to do some of the things that able-bodied people can do. A recent survey shows that approximately 15% of adults have some form of disability.

Disabilities may be present from birth, or they may be the results of accident or disease, which may require a change in lifestyle. However, an ever-increasing group of disabled people are those whose disability develops with age.

The main types of disability are as follows:

- difficulties in mobility

- impaired sight or hearing

- learning difficulties.

People with mobility difficulties may include patients with multiple sclerosis, spina bifida or injury, who are unable to walk and are confined to a wheelchair, or the elderly who walk slowly and awkwardly. People with learning difficulties also include those who have difficulty in reading or writing, which is still common.

Problems may arise when a person with a disability visits the surgery or hospital, and these may be due to the following:

- the premises

- the staff

- the patient.

Premises

Look at your place of work in a detached manner and imagine how it must be for a disabled person. Can a patient in a wheelchair readily gain access to the surgery premises or to your hospital department? Are there steps? Are the doors sufficiently wide for wheelchair access? Where can the wheelchair be placed in the waiting-area? Is there good light at the reception desk to aid lip-reading? Is there an area or room away from the reception desk where confidential matters may be dealt with, or for a private discussion with a deaf person? Are the notices clearly written and easy to read?

Staff

Empathy is the most important quality for any staff dealing with patients, but especially when dealing with disabled patients. Staff should be aware of the disability and anticipate what the difficulties may be. For example, sitting in a waiting-room and worrying that a call may be missed makes a deaf person very anxious. Secretaries and receptionists should be tactful and relate to the patient, help with the difficulties caused by the disability and allow more time to deal with their special needs.

Patients

You will find that the majority of patients with a disability are usually less demanding than many other patients. They try to be as independent as possible, although they are very much aware that special allowances may have to be made because they may be slower, or require things to be written down for them or, if they are in a wheelchair, they may take up more space in the waiting-area.

Secretaries and receptionists should be aware that some patients will try to hide their disability, and you should respect their wishes by offering advice without drawing attention to their problems.

Elderly patients

The medical secretary or receptionist should be aware of the many and diverse problems which may affect an elderly patient's access to healthcare, and try to minimise the effect of some of the following problems which may be encountered:

- impaired hearing
- impaired eyesight
- decreased mobility
- difficulty or inability to cope with new procedures
- reduced energy
- arthritic joints
- fear of being misunderstood
- fear of not understanding instructions

- a desire not to be a nuisance to doctors and staff

- socio-economic problems (e.g. financial problems, loneliness, increasing difficulty in day-to-day living).

Cultural issues and language barriers

Medical secretaries and receptionists should be able to identify an individual patient's ethnic or cultural needs and remember that their manner and the way in which they communicate with patients are important in ensuring that ethnic or cultural requirements are identified and met. Remember that if a patient is discourteous to you, it may be because they have difficulty in expressing themselves, or because they are worried about their medical condition. You should remain professional, polite and calm at all times.

Interpreters

Good communication plays a vital role in the provision of effective healthcare. Many patients, especially in inner-city areas, may have a very limited knowledge of the English language, and an interpreter may have to be used.

An interpreter may be available in some hospitals, or colleagues within the workforce may be able to help. On the other hand, interpreters are available from external sources and receptionists and secretaries should know how to contact them if it is felt that an interpreter may be of significant help in improving communication and understanding.

Patients may be accompanied by a relative or friend who is more fluent in the English language, when attending surgery or a hospital clinic, in order to facilitate communication.

Remember that there are still many people in this country who are illiterate. You should be particularly aware and sensitive when offering your help, as they are often extremely embarrassed about this.

Staff working in general practice will no doubt have a list of interpreting services available locally, or will be able to obtain information from their local authority social services department.

The decision as to which is used will depend on the purpose for which the interpreter's services are required.

External interpreters should be used:

- for formal communications (e.g. interviews, complaints procedures, etc.)

- if requested by the patient, relative or fellow professional involved in the care of the patient

- if professional services are deemed to be necessary to enhance understanding.

Visually impaired people

Guidelines are available from the Royal National Institute for the Blind (RNIB) for the provision of a 'user-friendly' environment for people with poor eyesight. These guidelines give suggestions for improving visibility and for providing tactile and auditory clues.

Visibility

Appropriate lighting is the most important aid to vision. People with visual impairment will need twice the quantity of light that is required by sighted people. As people get older, the need for effective lighting increases. The decor of the surgery or hospital should reflect the needs of people with impaired sight, and the use of contrasting colours will reduce disability. Shiny surfaces create reflection and glare, and if possible their use should be avoided. Obstructions must be kept to a minimum and highlighted. Be aware of potential hazards to the visually impaired, including the following:

- furniture
- planters
- toys left on the floor.

Ideally, all edges to furniture and walls should be rounded to minimise injury in the event of a collision. Signs and notices should be clearly written to be effective.

Any auditory clues that may be used must be direct, useful and readily understood.

Tactile clues and texture contrasts can be underfoot or at a suitable height for hand/finger touch, enabling the visually impaired person to identify a particular area, etc.

All staff who have contact with visually impaired people can do much to facilitate their access to healthcare.

- Ensure that all instructions are clear and readily understood.
- If necessary, take the person to a seat (they may not be able to see it), and then guide their hand to touch the seat or the back of the chair.
- Take them to the doctor's consulting-room, or to the nurse.
- Arrange help if they need to go from one hospital department to another.
- Help patients with poor eyesight to fill in forms, and if they need to sign their name, place their finger on the place of signature.

- When addressing the patient, use their name or touch them so that they know you are talking to them and not someone else. When you leave them, don't forget to tell them, so that they do not continue a conversation with someone who is not there.

- Use speech appropriate to people with impaired sight.

- Make sure that they are sitting safely, and that the doctor or nurse can see them.

People with hearing difficulties

Patients who have hearing difficulties or who are totally deaf may wish to communicate in writing, so make sure that you have a supply of pens and paper available. Perhaps some members of staff may be able to use sign language.

If you are dealing with appointments, it is a good idea to make a note in the appointments book of any such patients, so that they are not overlooked when their name is called out and so miss their appointment.

The following points will help you to communicate effectively with people who have hearing difficulties.

Face to face

- Speak up, but do not shout.
- Speak a little more slowly than usual.
- Maintain eye contact.
- Ensure that your face is well lit.
- Make sure that the person can see your face clearly to help lip-reading.
- Do not look away from the person when you are talking to them.
- If you cannot get the message across, write it down.

Telephone

- Speak up, but do not shout.
- Speak more slowly than usual.
- If the patient does not understand you, do not repeatedly use the same words, but instead rephrase what you are saying.
- When giving letters, use letters of the alphabet to clarify ('A' for apple, 'C' for Charlie, etc.).
- When giving numbers, appointment dates, etc., always ask the person to repeat them to ensure that they have understood.

People with learning difficulties

Staff working in both general practice and hospitals will find that they are dealing more and more with people with learning difficulties, who are now living in the community and have the same access to healthcare as anyone else. It is important that they are treated in precisely the same way, but making allowance where necessary to ensure that they get the best out of the health service. Therefore:

- be patient
- do not be intimidated – frustration at being unable to make themselves understood may make people with learning difficulties appear aggressive
- stay calm
- ignore any strange mannerisms and comments
- speak in simple, straightforward language.

Remember that there are still patients who are illiterate and who experience problems in accessing healthcare, perhaps when telephoning for an appointment for pathology or the antenatal clinic, for example. Although they may not be able to read what is written down, they may well be able to name individual letters, so be patient and ask them to give you the letters that form the written word, rather than subjecting them to the embarrassment of admitting to you that they are unable to read.

Children

Many children each day attend their doctor's surgery, the local hospital or community clinic. Everything should be done to provide for children's needs, including the following:

- a play area
- sturdy toys
- colourful books
- a changing area for babies and toddlers.

Again, if possible, chairs and tables in waiting-areas should have rounded corners to prevent serious injury.

Children are often frightened by a surgery or hospital, so staff should be sensitive to the special needs of children and do all that they can to provide a safe, reassuring and friendly environment.

In 1993 the Audit Commission published a report, entitled *Children First,* on the care of sick children. The report examined six principles of care and gave guidance as to how each of these should be adopted.

- *Child and family-centred care* – hospitals should be sensitive to the special needs of children and their families when in hospital, placing as much emphasis on the care and support of the child (which means the involvement of parents in their care) as on their medical needs. Services also need to be tailored to the wide age range of children (from under one year up to 18 years of age).

- *Specially skilled staff* – children should only be cared for by staff who are specially trained to meet their particular needs.

- *Separate facilities* – children should only be cared for in facilities which have been designed with their needs in mind. Where separate designed facilities do not exist, children should not be treated in other parts of a hospital.

- *Effective treatments* – children should only receive treatments which are known to be effective.

- *Appropriate hospitalisation* – children should only be admitted to hospital when the treatment and care cannot be provided in an alternative environment (e.g. in their home).

- *Strategic commissioning* – purchasers should be commissioning the types of service which most closely meet children's needs, particularly the development of hospital-at-home services to avoid hospitalisation as far as possible.

The National Association for the Welfare of Children in Hospital (NAWCH) has added to these principles in its Charter for Children in Hospital.

Working people

General practitioners and hospitals alike are becoming aware of the need to improve access to healthcare for working men and women by offering appointments at times that are better suited to their working hours. As a result, surgeries and clinics are offering appointments earlier in the morning, later in the evening, or reserving the first appointments for business people. Similar consideration is being given to mothers with children at school and to the elderly, by offering appointments at appropriate times during the day.

Transport

Patients with their own transport

Many patients will attend both hospital and general practice by car, and although hospitals are now providing more car-parking facilities for all patients, special consideration should be given to the elderly or those with physical difficulties by providing parking facilities as near as possible to the clinic that they are attending.

Similarly, although surgeries may not have the space to provide adequate parking for all patients, special consideration should be given to the elderly and patients with special needs to provide ease of access to healthcare.

Patients using public transport

Receptionists should be able to inform patients about local bus and train services, and to direct them to the appropriate pick-up/drop-off points to enable them to reach their destinations. Information about local taxi services should also be available to patients.

Patients using the ambulance service

Receptionists should be aware of the categories of patients who are eligible for transport by ambulance to and from hospital (walking with assistance, sitting or stretcher cases). Eligibility is assessed by general practitioners or social services, and receptionists will usually be asked by the GP to arrange appropriate transport for the patient's first visit to hospital. Subsequent transport for hospital attendance may be arranged by the hospital receptionist or secretary, but may also be arranged directly by the hospital's ambulance service administrator.

Total quality in medical practice

The phrase 'total quality' is frequently used without any definition of what total quality actually means for the organisation concerned.

NHS trusts, health authorities and GPs are concerned to provide a quality service to their patients (customers), and many of them are committed to a total quality programme. An appropriate definition of total quality in providing healthcare might be as follows:

a cost-effective system for integrating the continuous quality improvement efforts of all involved in healthcare to deliver services which ensure patient (customer) satisfaction.

Box 2.4 What is total quality?

Total quality strives to create a climate for excellence.

Total quality strives to prevent errors rather than to correct them.

Total quality is based on effective and harmonious teamwork with the absolute commitment of all members of the team.

What is a doctor's view of quality?

What is the patient's view?

What is your view?

Patients want easy access to a doctor either in hospital or in general practice. They would prefer to wait in pleasant surroundings and they want as short a waiting-time as possible. They want a reasonable amount of time set aside for their consultation, and they expect receptionists and secretaries to smile, and be sympathetic and responsive to their needs.

A doctor's perception of quality is probably very different, but they too expect an efficient service from their clerical staff as well as from the medical team in providing patient care.

Receptionists, secretaries, nurses and other members of the healthcare team all have different perceptions of quality. They cannot be expected just to provide an 'excellent' service while auditing themselves. They must be given the opportunity to share in the vision of what the organisation is attempting to achieve. To do the job well, everyone will need guidelines. Clear goals and objectives must be set and regular reviews and training given to help them to create the climate for excellence.

Team members will be encouraged to set their own objectives and to monitor and improve their individual performance. They should be able to make suggestions for improved working methods and to discuss new ideas for improving the service.

Total quality is an extension of customer care, in which every receptionist and secretary working in the field of healthcare plays a vital role.

Customer care: involving patients and the public

As a receptionist or secretary you may be involved in using questionnaires or short interview surveys to gather information, views and suggestions from patients and the public to provide an opportunity for them to express their opinions or decisions about healthcare or about local health service provision. Surveys are often designed at different levels:

- for patients and their own healthcare
- for patients and the public about the range of services
- when organising and planning service developments

(*Source*: Chambers R (2000) *Involving Patients and the Public*. Radcliffe Medical Press, Oxford.)

The NHS regards user and public participation as an important priority for all primary care groups, and believes that users of the NHS should have a greater voice and influence.

A national survey of NHS patients that has already been conducted confirms that patients want a fast and convenient health service, which is more in tune with the needs of the modern world. It also shows that people want a certain level of change and modernisation, and the need to shape and deliver its services in the same way.

The NHS Plan aims to restructure the health service from the patient's perspective and to give the patient more information and choice and to protect them from poor-quality service. This reflects the results of the 2000 survey.

NHS Direct and walk-in centres are part of the Government's plan to provide a more patient-focused health service.

Receptionists and secretaries will therefore, from time to time, be asked to assist with medical practice or health department satisfaction surveys or patient surveys, by gathering or collating information. This is all part of the customer care policy of your organisation, which is designed to highlight areas where an improvement in patient service is indicated.

Developing your personal effectiveness

Being assertive

Being assertive means treating other people with respect, asking for what you want and not blaming others for what happens to you. It stems from taking an honest look at strengths and weaknesses and accepting them. Assertive behaviour can include some or all of the mannerisms listed in Box 2.5.

This type of behaviour makes other people feel good when they talk to you because you value them and accept their behaviour, and you are not crushed or threatened by rejection because you do not depend on others for approval.

Box 2.5 Assertive behaviour

Voice	Steady, firm Tone is mid-range, rich and warm Sincere, clear
Speech pattern	Fluent Emphasises key words Steady, even pace Moderate speed
Facial expression	Responsive, matching the feelings expressed Open Steady features Attentive Interested
Eye contact	Direct Maintained
Body	Relaxed Open hand movements (inviting to speak) Sits upright or relaxed (not cowering or slouching) Stands with head held up

---

Managing time

To be effective at work, good time management is essential. Box 2.6 identifies some of the problems of poor management of time, the causes, and some possible solutions.

Looking after yourself

There is greater pressure than ever before on healthcare staff to work to maintain and improve the health of the community that they serve. A variety of initiatives come immediately to mind – antenatal and postnatal care, family planning, child development and immunisation clinics, screening (well-man, well-woman, elderly), health promotion programmes for specific conditions (e.g. diabetes, hypertension, asthma), healthy eating and anti-smoking advice, and health education literature and posters.

In a more general sense, everyone knows, in theory at least, that they should take certain basic sensible steps to maintain a healthy lifestyle, but for this to become a reality each individual has to understand how they

Box 2.6 Time management

PROBLEM	CAUSES	POSSIBLE SOLUTIONS
Having too much to do	Unclear priorities	Check goals or tasks clearly with your manager and check priorities. Each day, decide on your priorities and stick to them
	Wanting to be directly involved with everything	Be selective, and delegate if you can
	Unrealistic time estimates	Recognise that everything takes longer than you think – add 20% to your estimates
	Overwhelming pressure and piles of paper	Do not confuse activity with effectiveness – just because you are busy this does not mean that you are working well. Try to get into a fixed daily routine with definite times for jobs such as sorting the post, filing, etc.
Inability to finish things	Lack of deadlines	Always set deadlines
	Lack of respect for your time and interruptions by others	Fix a regular time when you need to be left undisturbed. Arrange to divert telephone calls, and agree to accept colleagues' calls in return. Be sure that you know what you want to achieve so that you can communicate this to others
	Doing too many jobs at once	Do one job at a time. When you start a piece of work, try to finish it if you can. You waste time each time you have to go back to it, while you remember where you had got to. Be systematic, as then if you have to leave a job part finished, it will make it easier for you, or indeed anyone else, to pick it up again
	Wasting time	Handle telephone calls promptly and write messages down immediately. When you make calls, plan what you are going to say beforehand and have all the necessary information to hand

| Lack of overview and perspective | Know your priorities. Use your diary. Try to transfer responsibility for some of your work when taking on new jobs. Fix a specific time for any major jobs which should not be interrupted |
| | Impose deadlines on yourself and tell others about them |

can help themselves to avoid health problems. In doing this, they will also be contributing to their own personal effectiveness both at work and at home.

Whether you are a doctor, a receptionist, a secretary or a nurse, the message is clear. You will do no one a good service if you do not build in time for looking after yourself.

Paying attention to your own health means taking a hard look at those factors which are known to contribute to poor health, including smoking, drinking to excess and being overweight, and making a conscious effort to take exercise, eat healthily and take advantage of all of the health-screening checks that are available.

Handling stress at work

Most people when discussing their jobs would refer at some point to the amount of pressure that they are under at work. Hopefully this will not be a constant problem, and in fact many people claim to work better when under slight pressure. The problems arise when the pressure becomes too great or continues for a long time.

An awareness of the difference between pressure and stress is important. Generally speaking, stress does not produce a positive or energetic response, but is reflected by panic reactions, irritability, an inability to relax and difficulty with relationships. It is also well known and well established that stress can lead to a variety of medical problems.

Stress at work may have a number of causes. The job may require a great deal of effort, or rapid decision making, or its requirements may be ambiguous and therefore lead to competing demands. Unsatisfactory working conditions, inconsiderate bosses or supervisors, shift work and so on can all put pressure on an individual's ability to cope.

Stress is a fact of life and cannot be eliminated. Indeed, most people would quickly become bored if too few demands were placed on them. The key issue is therefore that of coping – that is, the response made by an individual who encounters a situation with a potentially harmful outcome. Most people employ an enormous number of ways of coping with diverse demands, and often different combinations of different types.

In general terms, there are two major functions of coping. One is to alter the situation causing stress, and the other is to deal with the emotion that the stress engenders. The extent to which an individual is able to deal with these two aspects depends on a variety of circumstances. However, the fact that they both have an impact in varying degrees can help both in understanding situations better and in developing coping strategies.

Flexibility is important. It is more effective to use a variety of coping skills than to use one specific response. It is therefore necessary to be cautious when taking on board any fixed ideas on how to cope. However, there are some general guidelines which can help you to think through the situation (*see* Box 2.7).

Box 2.7 Coping with stress

Know yourself and the way in which you react.

Relax.

Decide what is important.

Look for support from others.

Keep communicating.

Use a step-by-step, problem-solving approach.

Summary

In this chapter we have looked at the contribution made by both receptionists and secretaries in the health service in their dealings with patients, and their role in creating the first impression that patients have of the healthcare provided in both primary and secondary care.

Quality of healthcare provision and customer care go hand in hand to achieve ever-improving standards and patient satisfaction.

3

Communication

Introduction

Communication is the technical term for passing on information. Effective communication occurs when appropriate information is not only passed on, but is seen to be understood and acted upon. Therefore the skills of communication involve the following:

- listening to and understanding what the patient/doctor requires
- conveying appropriate information
- checking that the information has been understood
- checking that a suitable response has been or will be made.

Box 3.1

For the medical receptionist the responsibility of communicating with patients is:

to listen first

then to give appropriate information

to check by questioning that the patient understands

and to confirm by observing whether action will be or has been taken whilst maintaining confidentiality.

Listening

Listening involves not merely hearing the words that are said, but also hearing what is not said, using intuition, common sense and reading behaviour to obtain the complete picture. On the telephone this is more difficult because body language (*see* Chapter 2) cannot be seen. However, it is important to tune into variations in tone of voice. With patients who are well known this will be an almost automatic process, but with those who are new it is even more important to exercise perception in order to get off to a good start.

The receptionist is the key person in ensuring that information is conveyed between patients, healthcare staff, hospitals, general practices, drug company representatives, pharmacists, suppliers and health authorities/health boards – to name but a few! It is vital that all of the communication skills are used to best effect.

The receptionist needs to be skilled in all forms of communication – verbal, in written form on paper, or by electronic means – but the majority of a receptionist's time will be spent in verbal communication.

Box 3.2

DO	DON'T
Speak clearly	Eat or drink while speaking
Do one thing at a time – give 100% attention to each patient	Do two things at once (e.g. hunt for missing files, or work on the VDU while speaking to someone)
Use words carefully	Use slang or medical jargon to patients
Control conversations with patients – use open and closed questions	Allow the patient to keep you longer than is necessary
Be aware of your own tone of voice	Allow anger or frustration to show in your tone of voice

---

Use of questions in communicating

Awareness of the use of questions can help the receptionist to draw out patient needs or wrap up an unduly lingering conversation. Although a certain amount of questioning will be done automatically, or according to the practice/hospital policy, when difficulty is encountered, using the right questions will help.

The simplest classification of questions is that they can be open, closed or leading.

- *Open* questions ease the patient into giving the information that is required. For example, 'How can I help you?' encourages the patient to state their need (for an appointment, test result, etc.).

- *Leading* questions encourage the patient to make a decision by stating alternatives from which one needs to be selected. For example, 'Do you want the appointment on Monday or Tuesday?', to which the logical answer is one of the two on offer, or 'You want to give up smoking, don't you?', to which the expected answer is 'Yes'.

- *Closed* questions bring the conversation to a halt. For example, 'Shall I tell the doctor you need to speak to him?', to which the logical answer can only be 'Yes' or 'No'.

Box 3.3

OPEN QUESTIONS begin with the words	CLOSED QUESTIONS begin with the words
When . . . .?	Would you . . . .?
How . . . .?	Shall I . . . .?
Who . . . .?	Are you . . . .?
What . . . .?	Do you . . . .?
Where . . . .?	May I . . . .?

Note: This is why 'May I help you?' is a poor way to address someone when you really want to help them, because the instant answer is either 'No', which is difficult for a British person to say outright to someone they do not know, or 'Yes', but this does not help the person to formulate their requirement!

Methods of communication

Communication is the way in which we transmit information, knowledge, thoughts and ideas from one person to another or to a group of people. In any organisation, large or small, communication is important for the business to function effectively.

The four main methods of communication are as follows:

- the spoken word (direct – face to face)

- the written word (e.g. diagrams, posters, notice-boards, etc.)

- the use of telephone systems, including facsimile, answering machines, VDUs, email, etc.

- non-verbal communication (body language) (*see* Chapter 2).

Communication: internal and external

Communication may be either internal or external. The following are examples of written communication.

Written messages

Secretaries and receptionists are always conveying urgent and non-urgent messages from patients or other professionals. It is vital that the messages do not get mislaid and that appropriate action is taken. They should contain the following information:

- the date and time when the message is received

- the name, address and telephone number of the caller

- the name of the intended recipient of the message

- a clearly written and concise message

- the name or initials of the person taking the message.

Memorandum

A memorandum (memo) is an internal written communication which may be used to convey short messages and information either to individuals or to all members of the healthcare team. Your organisation will no doubt use a memorandum form which has several headings.

Notice-boards

Notice-boards can be used to convey information both internally to the organisation and externally to visitors. Notice-boards should be positioned so that they are readily visible and accessible to all who are expected to see the notices displayed. They should be kept up to date, and a member of the team will no doubt have responsibility for this.

White-boards

These are often used in organisations to display information relevant to the day. Hospitals and surgeries may display notices about clinics running late, or health promotion information, etc.

Leaflets and posters

Hospitals and surgeries alike have access to a vast quantity of health promotion material and health messages to patients. Managers will often give receptionists responsibility for displaying leaflets and posters, which should be shown in such a way as to give impact to the intended message.

Protocols and procedures

All healthcare organisations will provide written protocols to communicate to members of the team the procedures for the activities in which staff are involved. Written protocols contain standards of quality, and should be written so that all members of the team involved in the task fully understand the procedures and thus achieve their objectives.

External written communication

Letters remain the most widely used method of written communication. Secretaries will be trained to provide a high standard of letter writing.

Letters are used to communicate with health authorities, NHS trusts, health authorities, health boards, medical professionals and patients. For example, GPs write referral letters to hospital consultants, and hospitals send discharge letters and reports to GPs.

Computers now provide a networking facility linking hospitals, health authorities, laboratories and medical practices.

Report writing

Medical receptionists and secretaries may be asked to investigate a procedure or system that is not running smoothly, or to give an account of an event or incident which has occurred.

Reports are written on a given subject to:

- convey information and ideas
- sometimes convey recommendations.

The features of a good report are that:

- it is easily understood
- it is always clear
- it is as long as it needs to be, but no longer.

A report must be complete and accurate with regard to the information it conveys and, because a decision may be based on the report, it must be correct.

A logical structure for the type of report you may be asked to present would be as follows.

1   Introduction:

- subject heading or title
- terms of reference – what you have been asked to find out
- procedure – how you found this out.

2   Body of report:

- findings – what you have found out.

3   Conclusion:

- conclusions – your conclusion or diagnosis
- recommendations – what you think should be done.

Medical receptionists and secretaries may be asked to type more detailed reports, some of which may require a formal business format. There will no doubt be a 'house-style' which should be used, otherwise reference to a manual of basic secretarial skills will give the necessary guidelines.

Note: A report must be accurate, clear, concise and logically arranged. It should be concise to the extent that there is no 'padding' or irrelevant detail.

Electronic mail

Electronic mail or email has become very much a part of our means of communication, both in our private lives and in the workplace.

It is an important and useful communication tool, as it allows us to communicate information, or to leave messages for our colleagues and professional people countrywide and all over the world, 24 hours a day.

Email allows the speedy and efficient transmission of information, enabling decisions to be reached more quickly and thus contributing to a more effective service.

Mobile phones: text messages

Healthcare professionals can usually be contacted by mobile phone, either directly or by leaving a 'voicemail' message or sending a text message. New technology is making it easier to contact healthcare professionals in times of emergency and to communicate details of any important developments or changes.

Pagers are, of course, still commonly used in most NHS organisations to contact NHS professionals when there is an emergency.

Telephone skills

Telephone callers only have tone of voice and words to go upon. Any frustrations that are felt at the time of answering the phone will be conveyed to the caller in the tone of voice and intonation of the words.

It is difficult to illustrate this point from the written word. However, consider the common phrase used by many organisations to answer the telephone: 'How can I help you?'. This can be said with genuine interest, conveyed by a warmth of tone. Alternatively, it can be said in a robotic tone which makes the caller feel as if they want to leave a message on an answer-machine for someone else to call back later!

Understandably, by 10.30 am on a busy Monday morning it may be difficult for a stressed receptionist to make an incoming caller feel 'welcome' – difficult, but not impossible. It may be helpful to have some kind of personal motto to say to yourself at difficult times, such as 'Do as you would be done by' or 'Speak as you would want to be spoken to'. Self-control, conscious use of a warm tone of voice, and the personal motto are useful aids to ensuring that the telephone is answered to a consistently high standard.

Telephone enquiries

Secretaries and receptionists receive numerous telephone enquiries during the course of their day-to-day work. They may be typing lengthy reports, running a busy surgery or clinic or retrieving data from the computer, but the telephone enquiries and requests continue! Maintaining the balance between conflicting demands is part of the job, and the telephone caller should never have the impression that you are too flustered or annoyed at being interrupted and too busy to deal with their request.

• Answer the telephone as promptly as possible.

• Announce the name of the practice or clinic, and give your name (you will no doubt have your protocol for this).

• Establish the caller's identity and try to help.

• If the caller is using a pay-phone, take the number and ring them back promptly if necessary.

• Politely ask the caller to hold if you need to deal with a visitor.

Golden rules when using the telephone

• Be polite.

• Do not eat while you are speaking on the telephone.

• Do not hold two conversations at the same time.

• Return to the caller every 30 seconds if you are keeping them on hold.

• If you are unable to help the caller yourself, track down someone who can – if necessary call them back.

People skills – face to face

In contrast to telephone communication, where the only indicators are words and tone of voice, in a face-to-face encounter there is the additional dimension of 'non-verbal communication'. This consists of the signals that are given out and picked up, sometimes subconsciously, but which cause a reaction every bit as strong as that to the words and tone of voice. For example, a patient who is failing to get what they want is not only likely to raise their voice, but may well lean forward over the reception counter. In response, the receptionist could either spontaneously lean forward with a matching aggressive reaction, step back from the desk in a defensive manner, or calmly remain in the same position. Not only does the body move and thereby speak more clearly than our words, but the hands and face highlight the expression of feeling. For example, hands may become clenched into fists and smiles disappear. With this knowledge in mind, the skill is to maintain self-control and gain control of the situation. There are no set patterns for dealing with difficult situations, but attending courses, practice in role play, watching video clips, discussing situations after they have occurred, watching colleagues and learning from their successes/ weaknesses can all contribute to gaining experience and improving existing skills.

The medical receptionist or secretary also needs constantly to bear in mind the fact that patients are likely to feel unwell, be anxious about what is going to be done to them and what the doctor may say, and concerned about the effect of their illness on their family. These feelings make patients stressed and therefore more sensitive to offhand treatment. From the moment they arrive, they need to feel that they are the one and only concern of the receptionist.

Box 3.4

Recall good and bad experiences of how you have been made to feel in shops, offices, hospital and the doctor's surgery.

What made you feel bad?

What made you feel good?

What can you incorporate into your way of working to make patients feel as good as they can in the circumstances?

Meetings

Staff meetings, departmental or primary healthcare team meetings and patient participation groups are the type of meeting where receptionists and secretaries may be required to express a view. With modern management techniques, meetings have become an important tool for communication. They provide the opportunity to find out what is going on, to be updated with the latest information and to contribute to forward planning. Even in a well-chaired, relatively informal meeting, staff who have every confidence in dealing with difficult patients at the desk may find it almost impossible to speak out with doctors and/or managers present. Skill in speaking out can be cultivated by practice and helped by planning.

Box 3.5

If you are going to be called upon to speak, prepare for the occasion.

DO

Read the agenda circulated a few days before the meeting.

Think about what you want to say.

Write down a few key words.

Define one statement that encapsulates your view succinctly.

Make an outline of what you want to say.

You should succeed in confidently making your point and gain respect not only for your view, but for your ability to communicate.

DON'T

Go into the meeting intending to say whatever comes into your head at the time.

You may lose the opportunity to express what you really want to say, waste other people's time, and lose their respect.

Performance review

Receptionists and secretaries will no doubt be aware of other forms of 'communication' within their organisations, such as performance review or 'appraisal' interviews, where they will be given the opportunity to discuss their personal strengths and limitations, and perhaps identify areas where further training is needed.

Counselling

Counselling may be defined as: 'assisting individuals towards independence or self-actualisation'. It is a form of communication that is designed to enable employees to make their own decisions or choices. It involves:

- listening
- guiding
- communicating
- information giving.

Counselling is non-judgemental, does not make assumptions, and can be used either to prevent a problem or to help to work through an existing problem.

The practice leaflet

Practice information leaflets communicate to patients the services available at the practice and how they may make better use of the primary healthcare service. New patients will find the practice leaflet a valuable source of information, not only about the services offered but also about the members of the primary healthcare team, the times of the surgery and clinic sessions, and how to contact the doctor in an emergency.

Your practice leaflets should be attractively designed to make both patients and potential patients aware of the services and quality of care provided. They should be prominently positioned on the reception counter and readily accessible to all callers.

Hospital information leaflets

NHS trusts and private hospitals and clinics will provide information about the services which they offer. As well as basic information about hospital clinics, open-access facilities and times of visiting, etc., they will give details of transport to the hospital and car-parking facilities.

Networking

Every organisation is changing to a greater or lesser degree on a regular basis. Staff come and go, the organisational structure changes, and responsibilities are shifted from one department to another. Therefore it is important that personal contacts are made and maintained so that if a receptionist/secretary does not know how to do something or does not have a vital piece of information, then there is always someone to turn to who will either know the answer themselves or 'know a man who does'. It is also important to keep up to date with the latest information by reading magazines as a vital supplement to networking.

Barriers to communication

Physical barriers

Physical barriers to communication may include the following:

- too much noise
- insufficient privacy
- frequent interruptions
- physical handicap (e.g. deafness, blindness or stammer)
- the reception counter being either too high or too low
- telephone constantly ringing.

Receptionists'/secretaries' language

The language used when speaking to patients is a vital part of good communication. You must be aware of:

- using words (and jargon) that the patient cannot understand
- talking too quickly or too quietly
- talking with a strong accent
- confusing patients by giving them too much information.

Patients' language

Patients from ethnic minorities may have difficulty in understanding and speaking the English language. You may have a colleague who can speak their language, or an interpreter may be necessary.

Psychological barriers

You must be aware of the psychological elements which may form barriers to good communication. Patients may find it difficult to communicate for the following reasons:

- feelings of inadequacy

- lack of confidence

- being emotionally upset by pain and/or anxiety about their medical condition

- being unable to concentrate because of illness or medication.

Attitudes of secretaries and receptionists

Remember the importance of positive non-verbal signs. A negative attitude will be a barrier to communication, for example:

- being impatient and rude

- not giving your undivided attention

- appearing critical or demonstrating a superior attitude

- avoiding eye contact

- appearing to be too busy

- feeling irritated and under stress.

Attitudes of patients

An understanding of the reasons for patients' attitudes may help you to deal with them in a sympathetic manner and to overcome the barrier that their attitude may present. For example, they may be:

- too ill to concentrate

- resentful at having to present themselves at the reception desk

- terrified that they may have a serious illness

- afraid of appearing stupid to the efficient secretary or receptionist

- struggling with a personal problem

- inhibited by finding that they know the receptionist or secretary socially.

Overcoming the barriers

An awareness of the barriers, combined with good common sense, is a good start to overcoming any problems.

- Try to answer all questions in a positive way.

- A pleasant manner, a smile and understanding often do the trick – it is hard to be difficult when empathy is extended to one.

- Always be polite.

- Be alert to any problems which might occur.

- Always try to be helpful, smiling, calm and able to cope.

- If patients are kept waiting for longer than is necessary, apologise and give an explanation.

- When making appointments, ensure that the patient has the date and time written down to avoid any future misunderstanding.

- Try to give each patient your attention when dealing with them. Make eye contact and listen carefully to what they are saying.

- Never sound tired or bored, or look as if you are not listening.

Confidentiality

Remember that the rules of confidentiality that apply to working in any healthcare environment are just as important when communicating with patients.

All information is privileged information, and *must not* be divulged without the doctor's prior consent.

4

Law, ethics and medicine

Introduction

The relationships between professional healthcare workers and between them and their patients are governed by the professional ethics and etiquette of medicine which have developed over the centuries, together with developments in medicine itself. Secretaries and receptionists working closely with doctors and other healthcare workers, as well as being in constant communication with patients, should be aware of the important role of ethics and etiquette.

Ethics relate to moral principles and standards of what is morally right and wrong, and are the guiding rules of professional behaviour. They are directed towards the benefit of the patients. *Etiquette* is concerned with the courtesy and politeness of normal behaviour.

History of ethics and etiquette

History shows that even from the earliest times, various legal systems have incorporated some degree of regulation of doctors. The earliest records were the Code of Laws of Hammurabi (1790 BC), when fees were regulated. Success was rewarded in accordance with the status of the patient, but failure was punished, frequently by mutilation.

The earliest record and declaration of ethics was made in the Hippocratic Oath (400 BC), which reflects the culture of the Hippocratic physicians. The standards expressed in the Hippocratic Oath, although no longer affirmed by today's physicians, are still accepted as the ideal of professional behaviour (*see* Appendix 2).

The Hippocratic Oath demonstrates the early concern of the profession to regulate itself by laying down basic standards of professional conduct, not only between doctor and patient, but also between teacher and pupil. For centuries thereafter, the principles of Christian humanism dominated the practice of medicine. Traditions of etiquette in public and private life gradually developed and, combined with the criteria of professional conduct, established the physician's position in society.

In 1798, the proposals of Sir Thomas Percival in Manchester ultimately became the *Professional Conduct of Physicians and Surgeons*, published in 1803. This laid down the foundations for modern ethical standards in the UK.

The Provincial Medical and Surgical Association that was formed in 1832, and which became the British Medical Association (BMA) in 1856, appointed a committee on medical ethics in 1849. This formed the basis of the General Ethical Committee of the BMA, which has always played a leading role not only in establishing ethical standards for the professional in the UK, but also in setting standards adopted as norms of conduct for doctors in many parts of the world.

The BMA was largely responsible for the establishment of the General Medical Council (GMC) under the Medical Act of 1858. The GMC has a regulatory role, and from time to time issues guidance to members of the medical profession to enable them to avoid action which might lead to charges of professional misconduct. (The roles of both the BMA and the GMC will be covered in more detail later in this chapter.)

Medical ethics and etiquette

Every medical receptionist and secretary must be aware of the important areas of ethical behaviour and etiquette. It has already been stated that ethics are directed towards the benefit of the patients, and many are bound into a code of conduct published by the GMC for doctors, and by other regulatory bodies for other health professionals. For example, the General Dental Council (GDC) maintains a register of dentists, and promotes high standards of dental education as well as standards of professional conduct among dentists. It also has disciplinary powers with regard to the professional conduct of dentists.

New regulatory bodies have been introduced for nursing, midwifery and health visiting and for allied health professions.

- In 2002 the Nursing and Midwifery Council replaced the UK Central Council (UKCC).

- The Health Professions Council includes groups of healthcare professions that were not previously covered by statutory regulation.

Key organisation: Council for Healthcare Regulatory Excellence

Formerly known as the Council for the Regulation of Healthcare Professionals, CHRE is a statutory body responsible to Parliament and independent of the Department of Health, It promotes best practice and consistency in professional self-regulation in nine bodies:
• General Medical Council
• General Dental Council
• General Optical Council
• General Osteopathic Council
• General Chiropractic Council
• Health Professions Council
• Nursing and Midwifery Council
• Royal Pharmaceutical Society of Great Britain
• Pharmaceutical Society of Northern Ireland
It has 19 members – one from each of the nine bodies and ten lay members. With parliamentary approval, CHRE can force the regulator to change rules. Ł It also has the power to refer unduly lenient decisions about professionals' fitness to practise to the High Court for review.

www.chre.org.uk

Figure 4.2   Council for Healthcare Regulatory Excellence.

• The Council for Healthcare Regulatory Excellence (CHRE) covers all of the other professional regulatory bodies.

The Nursing and Midwifery Council is the regulatory body which sets standards for the education and conduct of the nursing, midwifery and health-visiting professions. It also maintains the professional registers.

All regulatory bodies have the responsibility of maintaining the register of those allowed to practise as doctors, dentists, nurses, etc. The ultimate sanction on those judged to have behaved unethically is the removal of their names from the register, and thus the removal of their ability to practise.

There are no formal sanctions for those in breach of etiquette, but the rules have been established by custom. They aid communication between professionals and avoid damaging reputations, so they may be said to benefit patients indirectly.

A modern restatement of the Hippocratic Oath was formulated by the World Medical Association in 1947 to reflect the changing attitudes of society and major advances in medical science. It is known as the Declaration of Geneva:

I solemnly pledge myself to consecrate my life to the service of humanity;

I will give to my teachers the respect and gratitude which is their due;

I will practise my profession with dignity;

The health of my patient will be my first consideration;

I will respect the secrets which are confided in me, even after the patient has died;

I will maintain by all the means of my power, the honour and the noble traditions of the medical profession;

My colleagues will be my brothers;

I will not permit considerations of religion, nationality, race, party politics or social standing to intervene between me and my patients;

I will maintain the utmost respect for human life from the time of conception; even under threat I will not use my medical knowledge contrary to the laws of humanity;

I make these promises solemnly, freely and upon my honour.

There are four important areas of ethical behaviour and etiquette of which all secretaries and receptionists in medical practice should be aware, and the principles of which they should apply to their day-to-day work. These areas are:

- confidentiality
- trust
- confidence
- integrity.

Confidentiality

Confidentiality places a constraint upon all those who work in the field of healthcare. The terms and conditions of employment of medical secretaries and receptionists, wherever employed, will almost certainly contain a clause to the effect that any breach of confidentiality will result in disciplinary action, or even dismissal. They will no doubt be asked to sign statements signifying that this is fully understood.

The Declaration of Geneva maintains that a doctor must preserve secrecy in all that he or she knows – even after the death of his or her patient. However, there are certain exceptions to this:

- when the patient gives consent
- when it is undesirable on medical grounds to seek a patient's consent, but it is in the patient's best interests that confidentiality should be broken

- the doctor's overriding duty to society

- for the purposes of medical research, when approved by a local clinical research ethical committee or, in the case of the National Cancer Registry, by the Chairman of the BMA's Central Ethical Committee.

Doctors must be able to justify their decisions to disclose information. A doctor must ensure, as far as possible, that all medical information is kept in a secure place.

Confidentiality and medical records

Secretaries and receptionists are in the privileged position of having access to medical records which contain confidential information about patients, and they should always remember that patients trust doctors not to divulge any personal information which is contained in the records. Likewise, confidential information should never be discussed or divulged by secretaries or receptionists.

Discretion is necessary when dealing with enquiries from solicitors, relatives or representatives of the patient, and insurance companies. Staff should always be circumspect when they are dealing with patients. When speaking with colleagues, great care should be taken. Some hospitals insist that patients are referred to by their hospital number and not by their name.

Secretaries and receptionists working in a hospital will usually find that their medical records manager will require them to sign a form stating that they understand the legal and ethical aspects of confidentiality, and that any behaviour contravening this may result in termination of employment.

Any information that is contained in medical records may only be disclosed in certain circumstances.

Trust

As part of their work in dealing with patients and their families, doctors are entrusted with information that would not be divulged to others. Good medical practice is based on the maintenance of trust between doctors, patients and their families, with the knowledge that professional relationships will be strictly observed. Not only doctors, but also medical secretaries and receptionists must at all times exercise care and discretion to maintain this special relationship.

Confidence

Confidence, like trust, is also vitally important in the doctor–patient relationship. Staff should appreciate that if patients have been helped by a doctor on a previous occasion, they are confident that they will be helped in any further episodes. Although this may make the doctor's task easier, it also places added responsibility on him or her, as doctors know they cannot always succeed.

The trust and confidence which patients should ideally have in their physicians and surgeons provide them with the will to overcome illness and make a good recovery. It is important to appreciate that when people are ill they want to see doctors and their staff who treat them with kindness and consideration, and who respect their views and feelings.

Integrity

Doctors will act professionally and objectively in the best interests of their patients in their judgements and patient care. Receptionists and staff should also behave in a professional manner and remain circumspect at all times. Considerable pressure is placed on doctors and healthcare staff (e.g. by relatives, advertising, the media, etc.). It is perhaps worth considering the duties of a doctor and the rights of patients in the context of ethics and etiquette in medicine.

Doctors' duties

At the end of 1996, the GMC published *Duties of a Doctor*, which describes good medical practice and gives guidance on the duties of doctors registered with the GMC. Patients must be able to trust doctors with their lives and well-being. To justify that trust, they as a profession have a duty to maintain a good standard of practice and care and to show respect for human life. In particular, doctors must:

- make the care of their patients their first concern
- treat every patient politely and considerately
- respect patients' dignity and privacy
- listen to patients and respect their views
- give patients information in a form that they can understand
- respect the rights of patients to be fully involved in decisions about their care

- keep their professional knowledge and skills up to date

- recognise the limits of their professional competence

- be honest and trustworthy

- respect and protect confidential information

- make sure that their personal beliefs do not prejudice their patients' care

- act quickly to protect patients from risk if they have good reason to believe that they or a colleague may not be fit to practise

- avoid abusing their position as doctors

- work with colleagues in the ways that best serve patients' interests.

In all of these matters, doctors must never discriminate against their patients or colleagues, and must always be prepared to justify their actions to them.

Overall management

It is good medical practice for one doctor to be responsible for the overall management of a particular patient's illness.

Referral from a GP to a consultant has evolved in the patient's interest. A consultant or specialist should not accept a patient without referral from a GP, although there are exceptions (e.g. sexually transmitted diseases, family planning and casualty).

Consent to treatment

The patient's trust that their consent to treatment will not be abused is an essential part of their relationship with their doctor. For a doctor even to touch a patient without their consent constitutes an assault. Doctors offer advice, but it is the patient who decides whether or not to accept that advice. It is the doctor's duty of care to give advice about the significant facts and inherent risks to a patient, so that the patient understands the nature of the proposed treatment and is able to give their consent.

Patients' rights

Patients have certain rights with regard to their use of healthcare services. These rights generally fall into two categories:

1   the right to treatment
2   the right to confidentiality.

The right to treatment

All patients:

- have the right to be on a GP's list of patients

- have the right to see a GP (not necessarily their own doctor) at the GP's surgery at any time during surgery hours

- should have access to a telephone number at which a GP can be reached 24 hours a day, 365 days a year

- should be visited at home if it is considered necessary by the GP

- must receive any treatment which is immediately necessary when they are temporarily away from home

- have the right to change GPs without giving a reason, by applying to another GP

- have no absolute right to a second opinion, but the doctor should take reasonable care to seek one if they are unsure of the diagnosis or treatment

- need to give consent before being examined or treated

- are not legally bound to accept treatment. However, doctors can give essential treatment if the patient is temporarily incapable of understanding or consenting to treatment (e.g. due to alcohol or drugs). If the patient is permanently incapable due to mental illness, it is possible for a legal guardian to give consent

- have the right to refuse to be examined with a medical student present

- have the right to a full and truthful reply to any specific question unless the information may result in anxiety which could injure the patient's health

- have the right to see and amend medical records made on or after 1 November 1991, unless they will cause harm to the patient (*see* Access to Health Records Act 1990). Hospitals, private clinics, GP practices, etc. who hold patient information on computer have to conform to the Data Protection Act, which protects patients' rights (*see* Data Protection Act 1984)

- have the right to complain about their doctor if they have not followed their terms of service, or if a doctor behaves in an unethical manner.

The right to confidentiality

Doctors must not pass on information without the patient's consent except to those involved in their treatment and care or, when it is in the best interests of the patient, to close relatives. The law requires doctors to give information about patients to health and other authorities in the following circumstances:

- when ordered by a court
- if the patient has certain infectious diseases or food poisoning
- if they suspect that the patient is addicted to a 'hard' drug
- if they arrange an abortion for a patient
- if required by the police to help to identify a driver suspected of motoring offences.

Chaperoning

All too frequently we hear about doctors being accused of indecently assaulting their patients, and doctors today are at risk from such accusations. The presence of a third person as a chaperone, usually a nurse, is a valuable insurance for the practitioner. However, there may be occasions when the doctor's secretary or receptionist will be asked to be present at the consultation, particularly in private practice when a nurse is not always available.

On some occasions, a chaperone is requested, particularly by an elderly woman or a woman from an ethnic minority (where removing a veil in the presence of a male person who is not a member of the family is an uncommon occurrence). Any requests, particularly of a cultural origin, should always be treated with great respect.

The presence of a chaperone for unaccompanied children or patients with a mental disorder is often requested, not only for the protection of the doctor but also in very exceptional circumstances for that of the patient.

It is considered that chaperones are advisable, but it may be that one is not always available when required. Doctors normally exercise their discretion when requesting a chaperone, and are naturally very cautious as patients of both sexes have made complaints of indecent assault, and these are not necessarily limited to allegations against a doctor of the opposite sex.

If you are not comfortable in the role of chaperone, you should let your colleagues know, so that someone else will be available should the need arise.

If the patient is emotionally upset or mentally disturbed when consulting a doctor, the presence of a chaperone not only protects the doctor but may also relieve the patient of some embarrassment and anxiety.

Consent to treatment

Patients' rights are an area of continuing concern for doctors and patients alike, particularly with regard to the controversial issue of 'informed consent'. As a medical receptionist or secretary, you should remember that doctors always require signed agreement from patients:

- before carrying out surgery and/or procedures

- prior to involving patients in clinical trials

- before publishing medical photographs or medical data, either in print or in data form.

Consent becomes *'informed consent'* when patients are made fully aware of the risks, consequences or alternatives of any such treatment or procedure, and the risks involved in signing any form of consent. Doctors and other health professionals should tell patients about the complications of the procedure and the likelihood of its success. It should be ensured that the patient fully understands the explanation and has the opportunity to ask any questions, close relatives being involved if necessary.

Consent is only valid if the patient understands what their treatment involves and agrees to it.

Patients may choose whether or not to take part in medical student teaching or medical research, and may refuse to consent to this.

The consent of both the woman involved in termination of pregnancy and the consent of the physician is no longer necessary.

Similarly, a partner's consent to sterilisation is not legally required, but in accordance with Department of Health recommendations, doctors will usually want to consult the partner.

Children and young people

Children aged 16 years and over can normally consent to their own treatment. Young children under the age of 16 years may be able to consent if they are sufficiently mature to fully understand what is being proposed. However, in some instances (e.g. termination of pregnancy) a doctor will also require parental consent.

The regulatory bodies and their role

The General Medical Council

The General Medical Council (GMC) was established under the Medical Act of 1858 with the purpose of distinguishing between unqualified practitioners or 'quacks' and qualified medical practitioners. The Medical Register was thus established, which contains records of medical practitioners and their qualifications.

The GMC licenses doctors to practise in the UK under the provisions of the Medical Act of 1983. Its purpose is to ensure that the public is served by doctors who have the qualities it expects, and to protect them from doctors whose conduct, professional performance or health places patients at risk (General Medical Council: *Protecting Patients, Guiding Doctors*).

One of the most important functions of the GMC is to protect patients and to guide doctors.

Functions of the GMC

- The GMC keeps a register of all medical practitioners who have obtained qualifying degrees, giving them licence to practise. The GMC publishes this register, providing the public with the names of doctors who have acquired the necessary medical qualifications and experience to equip them to practise in the UK.

- It keeps a separate register of those practitioners who have obtained higher degrees.

- It sets out standards of medical education.

- It is responsible for the publication of the *British Pharmacopoeia* (*BP*).

- It has an important regulatory role in that it issues guidelines to all members of the medical profession to enable them to avoid actions which might lead to charges of professional misconduct.

- It has a duty to administer discipline. It is to the GMC that the public and medical profession may make complaints about a doctor's behaviour.

- It has the power, if such a charge is proved, to temporarily suspend a doctor from practising or, if necessary, to remove their name from ('strike them off') the register.

Professional self-regulation has always been at the forefront of the NHS, giving patients the security of knowing that the medical professionals who care for them are competent. In recent years, Dr Harold Shipman's conviction for multiple murders of his patients and the Alder Hey Inquiry into the retention of organs of dead children without the knowledge or consent of their parents have both highlighted the need for reform.

The NHS Plan states that all regulatory bodies must reform, become smaller and have more patient and public representation. They should also have faster and more transparent procedures. The Government has insisted that all regulatory bodies develop common systems across the different professions, and that their agreed standards put patients' interests first – they should make improvements based on feedback from their representatives, the public and patients. Complains must be dealt with swiftly and thoroughly in a way that is responsive to the complainant, but that also deals fairly with the professional about whom the complaint is made.

Professional self-regulation includes setting clear standards and guidelines for deciding who should remain members of the medical profession and for assessing their fitness to practise. This includes registration, education, training, continuing personal development and revalidation. The General Medical Council is committed to maintaining public confidence and to responding to and protecting patients.

Following the Shipman Inquiry, the Government proposes to review the General Medical Council's role and system of revalidation, as well as the NHS's role in appraisal and assessment of a doctor's fitness to practise. It has proposed that it will introduce these arrangements in 2006 and that it will look at ways of modifying the General Medical Council's structure.

Changes have recently been made to disciplinary procedures for doctors and dentists which have abolished the distinction between personal and professional misconduct. NHS doctors and dentists will now face the same locally based procedures as all other staff. The employing trust is thus responsible for disciplining both medical and dental staff.

The British Medical Association

The British Medical Association (BMA) was founded in 1832 by Charles Hastings, and it is the largest medical association in the UK. It is concerned with most aspects of medicine and is one of the principal bodies representing UK doctors.

The BMA played an important part in the establishment of the General Medical Council. The Ethics Department of the BMA plays a leading role in establishing ethical standards in the medical profession. It examines and advises on the increasing number of ethical matters in medical practice, and on the relationship between doctor and patient. The BMA issues guidelines on various ethical issues including the following:

- euthanasia

- genetic counselling

- surrogacy.

The BMA publishes one of the world's leading medical journals, the *British Medical Journal*, which covers many topics of concern and interest to the medical profession, including original papers on clinical, scientific, political and social subjects.

Medical science is advancing rapidly and, with new discoveries being communicated to the public, the BMA issues ethical guidelines that reflect and safeguard the well-being and interests of patients, and at the same time express the views of the profession on medical ethics.

Summary of medical ethics and etiquette

In looking at the ethics and etiquette of medical practice, the medical receptionist or secretary will understand that patients expect doctors not only to use their expertise and skill, but also to observe absolute confidentiality with regard to any information that is imparted as a result of the consultation, examination and treatment. On this understanding of professional confidence and secrecy, all of those working in the field of healthcare will be aware of the special relationship which exists between doctor and patient.

Having considered the various ethical issues that confront the medical profession, and the role of the regulatory bodies, we are now able to appreciate the problems facing doctors and their ability to resolve the numerous ethical and moral dilemmas that may arise. These include the following:

- abortion

- euthanasia

- screening

- genetic counselling

- artificial insemination

- severely malformed infants

- *in vitro* fertilisation

- consent to operations on reproductive organs

- HIV/AIDS

- surrogacy

- transplantation

- the use of human tissue

- other issues arising from advances in biomedical and biological research.

Practical considerations for secretaries and receptionists

- Remember that your work is strictly confidential – anything that is divulged by a patient to the doctor, the medical records or correspondence, must not be disclosed to anyone else.

- Details of your work or personal affairs of doctors and other healthcare professionals must *not* be discussed.

- The behaviour of or treatment by a medical practitioner or any professional healthcare worker must *not* be openly criticised within hearing distance of the patient.

- Always be circumspect when talking about a doctor or other healthcare professional to another person. Do not unduly praise or criticise their accomplishments.

- It is your responsibility to facilitate the doctor's treatment and care of his or her patients.

Legal aspects

Medical secretaries and receptionists, although they do not need a detailed knowledge of law, should have an understanding of those legal aspects that affect their day-to-day work.

Patient access to information

Over the past decade, patients and carers have had an increasing expectation of access to information about their own healthcare, and this trend has been encouraged by NHS policy. There are very good reasons for giving patients access. First, it is ethical to do so, as truth-telling is not only a moral absolute but also produces a relationship based on mutual trust. Secondly, there is abundant evidence that people want more information about their own healthcare and treatment, and clinical trials have demonstrated that improved functional and health status is linked to good doctor–patient information sharing. Thirdly, legislation requires that patients should have access to information, and their rights to information in the UK (since 1991) were set out in the Patient's Charter, which summarised the rights and standards based on both legislation and common law. The right of access to health records was established by two acts of Parliament:

- the Data Protection Act 1984
- the Access to Health Records Act 1990.

More recently, new agendas have emphasised the need for improved patient access to information, including the following:

- Purchasing Intelligence and Local Voice
- NHS Code of Openness
- Patient Partnership Strategy
- Promoting Clinical Effectiveness
- NHS Research and Development.

There is an increasing awareness that sharing information with patients, carers and the wider public can be a significant factor in encouraging informed and discerning use of health services. Sharing information also encourages professionals to develop skills in communicating with patients.

The NHS Code of Openness (published in 1995) encourages both purchasers and providers to enable public access to information about NHS organisations, including trusts and health authorities and, patient advice and liaison services (PALS). The public also have the right to attend certain meetings of NHS organisations, and have the opportunity to put forward their views, as part of a commitment to public consultation. This includes information about costs, quality and performance, proposed service changes and how to influence decisions and actions that affect their own treatment, and what information is available and how to obtain it. There has been a recent noticeable growth in information services for patients and the public. Under the Patient's Charter, a single national freephone number for health information was established and health service guidelines required local centres to provide information on the following:

- common illnesses and treatments
- self-help groups
- waiting-times

- healthcare services
- keeping healthy
- patients' rights and how to complain
- Patient's Charter standards.

Medical records

NHS trusts, general practices and all healthcare organisations which record information on computer concerning identifiable living individuals must ensure that they comply with the provisions of both the Data Protection Act 1984 and the Freedom of Information Act 2000.

The Data Protection Act 1984

The Data Protection Act is designed and based on principles to ensure that information relating to an individual is obtained fairly, kept up to date and stored securely. Individuals whose data are stored have rights of access enabling them to check the accuracy of the information. The data protection registrar and the courts are empowered to require correction of inaccurate material if it is not undertaken voluntarily by the data user.

The medical context of the individual's right of access to information held about him or her has been modified by the Data Protection (Subject Access Modification) (Health) Order 1987. This allows information to be withheld from an individual if it is likely to cause serious harm to his or her mental or physical health, or if it discloses the identity of a person other than the healthcare professional. A doctor who withholds information must be prepared to justify his or her actions in a court if challenged at a later date. This Act applies to England, Wales, Scotland and Northern Ireland.

Freedom of Information Act 2000

The Freedom of Information Act requires every public authority to adopt a 'publication scheme' that specifies the classes of information which the authority publishes, the form it takes and whether it charges for the information. Each scheme must be approved by the Information Commissioner, an independent public official who is responsible for overseeing operation of the Act and who also has powers of enforcement.

Since January 2005, NHS organisations have been obliged to answer requests for information within the terms of the individual right of access given by the Act. This applies to all recorded information held by the organisation regardless of its date, although the Act specifies some exemptions. Anyone making a request must be told whether the organisation holds the required information and, if it does so, they must be supplied with it (generally within 20 working days). Organisations also have a legal duty to provide advice or help to anyone who is seeking information. If a request for information is denied, it may be possible to appeal against the decision.

Further information can be found at www.informationcommissioner. gov.uk

The Access to Medical Reports Act 1988

This Act establishes an individual's right of access to medical reports prepared for insurance or employment purposes by doctors who either are, or have been, responsible for that person's care. The Act applies only to England, Wales and Scotland, but similar provisions now apply to Northern Ireland under the Access to Personal Files and Medical Reports Order 1991.

At the same time that the patient's consent to the preparation of the report is obtained, the commissioning company is required to inform the individual of his or her rights under the Act, and to enquire whether access to the report is required. The information is then passed on to the doctor.

If the patient requires access, he or she is allowed 21 days to make appropriate arrangements to view the report. Patients who originally declined the opportunity of access may make an application to see the report until the time it is despatched to the company and, if so, must be allowed 21 days to make appropriate arrangements.

Once the report has been seen by the patient, he or she may agree to the despatch unaltered, request correction of factual accuracy or, if the doctor declines to make the requested correction, append a statement of their own, or they may refuse to allow the report to be released.

The Human Rights Act 1988

The Human Rights Act incorporates the European Convention on Human Rights (ECHR) into English law. It brings with it new responsibilities for all who work in public authorities. Our courts now have to take into account the case law of the European court.

The main aim of the Act is to allow the rights given under the European Convention on Human Rights (ECHR) of 1950, and the Act will contribute towards a society where the rights and responsibilities of individuals are carefully considered and where awareness of the rights of the ECHR permeate government and legal systems.

A 'public authority' includes the following:

- central government
- local government
- the courts
- police.

It also includes many other bodies who carry out functions which the Government would otherwise have to undertake, including health authorities and trusts, local authorities, government agencies, courts and tribunals. Any person or organisation that carries out some functions of a public nature is also included, although under the Act they are only considered to be a public authority in relation to their public functions.

All public authorities have a positive obligation to ensure that respect for human rights is at the core of their day-to-day work, which means that they should act in a way that positively reinforces the principles of the Act. This is further emphasised by the fact that it is unlawful for a public authority to act (or fail to act) in a way which is incompatible with an ECHR right. This includes the following aspects of the activities of a public authority:

- drafting rules and regulations

- internal staff and personnel issues

- administrative procedures

- decision making

- policy implementation

- interaction with members of the public.

At the very core of every organisation there should be respect for ECHR rights, and if existing procedures are not compatible, new policies and procedures will have to be implemented.

In their day-to-day work, public authority officials should always act in accordance with the ECHR rights in demonstrating a positive attitude to human rights.

The Access to Health Records Act 1990

This Act applies to England, Wales and Scotland and has established a right of access for patients to whom the records relate and, in certain circumstances, to other individuals. The Act also makes provision for correction of inaccurate records.

Under the Act, a health record is any record containing information relating to the physical or mental health of an individual who can be identified from that information which has been made by 'or on behalf of' a healthcare professional.

Applications for access must be made in writing to the record holder and, provided that no addition to the record has been made within the previous 40 days, a fee may be charged. Provided that there is no reason to withhold access, the record holder must allow the applicant to see the records within 40 days, unless the most recent note has been made within 40 days, in which case the time limit is 21 days. If a copy of the medical record is required, a copying and postal charge may be made. Applications may be made by the patient or by someone appointed on the patient's behalf. This may be:

- in the case of a child, the parent or guardian

- in the case of an incapable patient, a person appointed by the court to manage the patient's affairs

- after a patient's death, the patient's personal representatives or anyone who might have a claim arising out of the patient's death.

The law and mental health

Mental Health Act

Secretaries and receptionists working in the field of healthcare will need an understanding of the implications of the law relating to mental illness.

The law changed with the Mental Health Act of 1983. The provisions of this Act are of particular importance to those patients who are compulsorily detained under the Act. This involves approximately 10% of all patients who are admitted to psychiatric hospitals or departments.

The Mental Health Act of 1983 established the Mental Health Act Commission, which has a responsibility to protect the rights of detained patients and to keep under review the exercise of compulsory power and duties conferred by the Act. The Act also provides the legal instrument which enables society to act in the interests of, and on behalf of, patients and those convicted of certain criminal offences who are diagnosed as having certain abnormal mental conditions, and makes provision for the protection of the public, and for the protection of the property of patients who are compulsorily detained.

The primary concerns of the 1983 Mental Health Act are:

- protection of the mentally ill patient
- protection of his or her property
- protection of the public.

The Act defines certain relevant legal mental conditions as follows.

- *Mental disorder* – which means illness, arrested or incomplete development of mind, psychopathic disorder or any other disorder or disability of mind.

- *Severe mental impairment* – which means a state of arrested or incomplete development of intelligence and social functioning, and is associated with abnormally aggressive or seriously irresponsible conduct on the part of the person concerned.

• *Mental impairment* – which means a state of arrested or incomplete development of mind (not amounting to severe mental impairment) which includes significant impairment of intelligence and social functioning, and is associated with abnormally aggressive or seriously irresponsible conduct on the part of the person concerned.

• *Psychopathic disorder* – which means a persistent disorder or disability of mind (whether or not it includes significant impairment of intelligence) which results in abnormally aggressive or seriously irresponsible conduct on the part of the person concerned.

A person may not be regarded as suffering from mental disorder by reason only of promiscuity or other immoral conduct, sexual deviancy or dependence on alcohol or drugs.

The legislation emphasises the following:

1   as much treatment as possible on a voluntary basis, both in hospital and in the home or other institution
2   a shift from institutional care to care within the home as far as is possible
3   proper provision for those to be detained on a compulsory basis in the interests of the patient and society.

Medical secretaries and receptionists will from time to time be involved in arrangements for patient admission, either formally or informally, to undergo psychiatric treatment. Such admissions come within sections of the Mental Health Act. A brief outline of admission under some of the sections of the Mental Health Act is given below.

Methods by which a person may enter a hospital for psychiatric treatment

Informal admission (Section 131)

Any person having attained the age of 16 years may request admission, or a person under the age of 16 years where the parent or guardian gives consent, or any person to whom it is suggested that admission is advisable and that person does not refuse, can be admitted without any legal formalities. This patient can discharge him or herself unless the doctor in charge decides that, if discharged, he or she would be endangering his or her health or safety or that of others.

Compulsory admission and detention

The following methods of admission can be used when a person suffering from mental disorder as defined by the Act is in need of psychiatric care but is not prepared to enter hospital or remain in hospital for observation or treatment.

- *Section 2 (up to 28 days)*: Admission for assessment (or for assessment followed by medical treatment).
  An application for the admission of the patient must be made by either an approved social worker or the nearest relative, plus a medical recommendation from one 'psychiatrist' and a doctor (if practicable, one doctor should have previous acquaintance of the patient – for example, his or her GP). The person making the application should have seen the patient within the last 14 days.

- *Section 3 (up to six months)*: Detention for treatment.
  The application for detention under Section 3 is the same as that for Section 2, except that the approved social worker is not to act if the nearest relative objects. This section can be reviewed for a further six months, and yearly thereafter.

  Note: Patients may apply to the Mental Health Review Tribunal (MHRT) under Sections 2 and 3, subject to the stated criteria.

- *Section 4 (up to 72 hours)*: Admission for assessment.
  The application must be made by either an approved social worker or the nearest relative, plus a recommendation from a medical practitioner who must have seen the patient within the last 24 hours. The patient must arrive at the hospital within 24 hours of the medical examination. (This may be converted into Section 2 if a second medical recommendation is received within 72 hours.)

Consent to treatment

Certain sections (56–64) of the Mental Health Act are largely concerned with consent to treatment for long-term detained patients, but certain safeguards also apply to informal patients.

The Mental Health (Patients in the Community) Act 1995

The Mental Health (Patients in the Community) Act 1995, which came into force on 1 April 1996, introduced a new power of supervised discharge available in the case of unrestricted patients who, in the opinion of the responsible medical officer, are ready to leave hospital but, because of the risk they present to themselves or others, need special support to live safely in the community. The patient's care plan, which must be in place before an application for supervised discharge is made, may include formal requirements such as attendance for rehabilitation or treatment, or the requirement to live at a particular residence. A named supervisor and responsible medical officer will be identified. Non-compliance will lead to an immediate review and possible compulsory readmission.

Care Programme Approach

The Care Programme Approach (CPA) is one of the cornerstones of policy on mental health, providing a framework for the care of mentally ill people which ensures that services are targeted at people with severe mental health problems.

Building Bridges

This paper, which was published in November 1996, offers detailed advice and guidance on arrangements for effective, co-ordinated, inter-agency work for the care and protection of severely mentally ill people.

Reforming the Mental Health Act

The White Paper published in December 2000, *Reforming the Mental Health Act*, describes the Government's proposals for legal reforms to reflect changes in mental healthcare, in particular the increased use of treatment in the community.

The White Paper is divided into two parts. Part 1, entitled *The New Legal Framework*, explains how new mental health legislation will operate for patients generally. It outlines the following:

- a new broad definition of mental disorder*

- a new three-stage process for the use of compulsory powers

- a range of safeguards for patients' interests, including a new independent Mental Health Tribunal, a right to independent advocacy, a new Commission for Mental Health, and a statutory requirement to develop care plans

- new duties covering the disclosure of information about patients who are suffering from a mental disorder.

*A new broad definition of mental disorder covers any disability or disorder of mind or brain, whether permanent or temporary, that results in impairment or disturbance of mental functioning. The same criteria will be used to determine whether an individual falls within the scope of the legislation, whatever their diagnosis.

Part 2, entitled *High-Risk Patients*, sets out specific arrangements for individuals who are deemed to pose a significant risk of harm to others as a result of their disorder. It outlines the following:

• new criteria linking the use of compulsory powers to the availability of a treatment plan needed to treat the underlying mental disorder
• the establishment of new facilities for those who are dangerous and severely personality disordered (DSPD).

Mental Health Bill

In 2005 the Government published its revised Mental Health Bill (which was severely criticised) in an attempt to reform the Mental Health Act 1983. The present Government will decide whether or not they will attempt to reintroduce it to Parliament.

Employment rights

There are a number of laws that influence the employment of staff. It is important that all employees, including medical secretaries and receptionists, understand their rights. Employees, and in some cases prospective employees, can seek compensation through an employment tribunal if employers do not comply. The key areas covered by legislation are noted at the end of this section in Box 4.1.

Written statement of main terms and conditions

From the point when a verbal offer of a job has been made and the post accepted, the formal contract comes into being. At this stage nothing further is required to signify its existence and both parties are bound by it from that point on. However, to avoid any misunderstanding, employers will generally follow up a job offer and acceptance with a letter.

Employers are required to provide all employees who are employed for more than one month with a written statement of the main terms and conditions of their employment within two months of starting work. All staff must be given notification of any changes to specified terms and conditions when they occur.

The written statement must contain the following information:

• employer's name
• employee's name

- the starting date of employment
- the date when continuous service began and whether or not employment with another employer (another hospital or medical practice) is counted
- job title
- rate of pay
- payment intervals (monthly, weekly)
- hours of work
- place of work
- holiday entitlement and holiday pay.

The following additional information must also be provided within the two-month period (as part of the principal statement or separately):

- sick leave and sick pay
- pension scheme
- notice periods on either side
- end date of a fixed-term contract, or likely end date of a temporary one
- particulars of collective agreements where these apply (e.g. Agenda for Change Terms and Conditions)
- grievance procedure and with whom a grievance can be raised
- disciplinary rules and procedures, and to whom appeals can be made.

Sometimes relevant information relating to sickness, pensions, grievances, disciplinary rules, procedures and appeals is kept in separate reference documents. In this case, the written statement will refer to these, and they should be readily accessible to employees in the course of their work.

Equality of opportunity

We discriminate between people both in the workplace and in day-to-day life. Some forms of discrimination are acceptable but others are not, and certain forms have been determined to be unlawful. Legislation relating to equality of opportunity requires employers to exercise some form of social responsibility in making decisions about current or potential employees. Employees, too, may unconsciously discriminate between people – we are not always aware of how our prejudices and preconceptions colour our judgement and the way in which we deal with others.

Equality can only be achieved through an acceptance by all members of the work team that it is important, in their own interests and in the interests of the service that they provide.

Equal opportunities legislation

Equality of opportunity regardless of sex, race, marital status, disablement, religion or age is vitally important, not only for employees to have a fair and equal chance of developing their potential abilities and realising their expectations, but also for employers to make full and effective use of their staff and to improve employee relations. This legislation forbids discrimination between men and women with regard to pay and other terms in their contracts. Examples are listed below.

1   *Equal pay*

Employers must provide equal pay for work of equal value. This includes:

- overtime
- bonus payments
- holiday and sick pay entitlements.

2   *Rehabilitation of offenders*

Employers are required to allow an individual who has had a conviction for an offence to put it behind them and be rehabilitated after a period of time. Their conviction becomes 'spent' and they may lawfully conceal it from a prospective employer as if it had never happened. However, certain exemptions exist.

3   *Sex discrimination*

Direct or indirect discrimination occurs if, on the grounds of her sex, a woman is treated less favourably than a man would be treated.

4   *Race relations*

Racial discrimination in both employment and the provision of services is unlawful. Legislation requires that no person should treat another less favourably on racial grounds, and places a duty on public bodies to provide equality of opportunity.

5   *Disability discrimination*

Legislation provides protection against discrimination for those who can show that they have a physical or mental impairment which has a substantial and long-term effect on their day-to-day activities. Employers are expected to make reasonable adjustments to the working environment where these will alleviate the disadvantages or risks faced by employees or prospective employees.

Sexual harassment

Sexual harassment is judged as unlawful behaviour contrary to the Sex Discrimination Act 1974. All supervisory staff are responsible for eliminating any sexual harassment, victimisation or intimidation of which they are aware. Examples of sexual harassment include the following:

- unwanted physical contact
- requests for sexual favours
- unwelcome sexual advances
- continued suggestions for social activity outside work after it has been made clear that such suggestions are not welcome
- offensive flirtation, suggestive remarks, etc.
- the display of pornographic or sexually suggestive pictures, etc.
- leering, whistling or making sexually suggestive gestures
- derogatory or degrading abuse or insults which are gender related
- offensive comments about appearance or dress.

Working-time regulations

These have been in place since 1 October 2000, and they provide new basic rights and protection for many workers, ensuring that they do not have to work excessive hours, and can take adequate breaks both within the working day and between shifts. In addition, they give rights to four weeks of paid holiday entitlement.

Part-time workers

From 1 July 2000 new regulations came into force for the purpose of ensuring that individuals in part-time employment are treated no less favourably than those in full-time employment.

Support for parents, families and carers

Legislation to support women in maternity has existed for many years and now extends support to parents and carers.

- *Time off for dependents* – all employees have the right to take a reasonable period of time off work in order to deal with an emergency involving a dependent.

- *Parental leave* – individuals who meet the conditions within the regulations may take up to 13 weeks' unpaid leave.

- *Maternity leave* – employees have the right to take maternity leave, receive maternity pay, and return to the same or a similar job.

Box 4.1 Areas covered by employment legislation and regulation

Contracts and statements of main terms and conditions

Discipline and grievance

Discrimination

Flexible working rights

Harassment and bullying

Health and safety

Maternity, paternity, adoption and parental rights

Record keeping

Redundancies and transfers

Termination of employment

Wages and salaries

Whistleblowing

Working time

Flexible working

Employees with children under six years of age (or under 18 years if disabled) may request flexible working arrangements if they are responsible for the child's care and have the necessary service. Their request must not be unreasonably refused.

Record keeping

Employers must comply with the requirements to hold, store, protect the confidentiality of and disclose records relating to staff.

Termination of employment

Employees with a year's service have the right not to be unfairly dismissed. If the dismissal was on grounds of discrimination, they do not need to have a year's service.

Whistleblowing

Employees are protected from incrimination if, after following the proper internal channels, they disclose genuinely held concerns.

Certification

All doctors, whether they are working in private practices or in an NHS organisation, are from time to time requested to issue certificates, including the following:

- National Insurance/DSS certificates
- death certificates
- cremation certificates
- private medical or insurance certificates
- certificates of stillbirth.

Certification is a statutory obligation that is imposed upon doctors, and the secretary or receptionist should do all that they can to ensure that the doctor is not placed in the position of being asked to certify improperly.

For example, the doctor must always see the patient when issuing and signing the form on which a patient claims sickness benefit – Form Med 3 and 5. This should not be issued more than one day after examination, as the doctor has to certify that he or she has examined the patient today/yesterday.

Death certificates

The death certificate is the oldest of all official medical forms and is only issued to registered practitioners. The certificate is obtained from the registrar for the subdistrict in which the doctor practises. The issue of death certificates is a statutory requirement and no fee is chargeable. The certificate is given by a doctor who was actually attending the patient in their last illness, and where there is sufficient knowledge of the cause of death to do so. Doctors are bound by law to provide the certificate in a sealed envelope. The death certificate should be taken to the Registrar of Births and Deaths in the subdistrict of occurrence within five days of death.

There is no legal duty to notify the coroner of any death, but of course this does not imply that the doctor need not do so when the circumstances require such action. Moral, ethical and traditional considerations necessitate that the doctor acts with responsibility and, by notifying the coroner, facilitates any enquiry into the death as the coroner deems advisable.

Role of the medical secretary or receptionist

Secretaries and receptionists must appreciate that when dealing with grieving relatives, sympathy, understanding and patience will be required. They should ensure that the death certificate is available when required, and clearly explain what the relatives/representatives should do with it (e.g. take it to the registrar's office within the statutory time, and, if necessary, give them directions).

Cremation certificates

Doctors may be requested to sign cremation certificates for patients they have attended during their last illness. Cremation certificates require confirmation by another doctor. Two signatures are always necessary, and a doctor may be asked to sign in either capacity. These certificates are available from local funeral directors, and the secretary or receptionist may be asked to ensure that there are forms available when required. A fee is payable to both signatories.

Private certification

Private certificates are issued to patients for purposes outside the scope of the NHS. They are used to supply information to organisations concerning proof of illness, such as the following:

- holiday insurance
- sick pay and superannuation purposes
- solicitors
- insurance companies
- schools.

A fee may be charged for private certificates. The BMA makes recommendations for fees, and doctors will charge according to their recommended scale.

Certificate of stillbirth

A doctor must sign a certificate of stillbirth if he or she was present at the delivery or examined the body of a stillborn child, and must give it to the person who will inform the registrar.

Birth registration

Every live birth or stillbirth must be registered within 42 days. It is the duty of either of the parents to register the birth. In the case of an illegitimate child, the duty to register the birth rests with the mother.

All certificates should either be stamped with the doctor's name, address, etc. or be printed in the case of a private certificate.

The Local Medical Officer must be notified of all births, either by the hospital or by the doctor in attendance.

Abortion certificates (termination of pregnancy)

The law in the UK allows doctors to terminate pregnancies as long as certain conditions are met:
1   two doctors must see the patient
2   they must agree that the conditions laid down in the 1967 Abortion Act have been satisfied.

Note: These conditions allow doctors to recommend termination when they feel that to continue with the pregnancy would be a hazard to either the physical or mental welfare of the pregnant woman or to any existing children of her family.

Secretaries and receptionists may be responsible for ensuring that the appropriate certification forms are available when required (*see* Figure 4.2).

Health and safety at work

The legislation relating to health and safety at work is complex, and although they are not directly responsible for workplace standards, medical secretaries and receptionists should be aware of the implications of the Health and Safety at Work etc. Act 1974 and of their personal responsibilities.

IN CONFIDENCE   **CERTIFICATE A**

ABORTION ACT 1967

Not to be destroyed within three years of the date of operation

**Certificate to be completed before an abortion is
performed under Section 1(1) of the Act**

I, ...
(Name and qualifications of practitioner in block capitals)

of ....

....
(Full address of practitioner)

Have/have not* seen/and examined* the pregnant woman to whom this certificate relates at

....

....
(full address of place at which patient was seen or examined)

on ....

and I ....
(Name and qualifications of practitioner in block capitals)

of ....

....
(Full address of practitioner)

Have/have not* seen/and examined* the pregnant woman to whom this certificate relates at

....

....
(Full address of place at which patient was seen or examined)

on ....

We hereby certify that we are of the opinion, formed in good faith, that in the case

of ....
(Full name of pregnant woman in block capitals)

of ....

....
(Usual place of residence of pregnant woman in block capitals)

(Ring appropriate letter(s))	A	the continuance of the pregnancy would involve risk to the life of the pregnant woman greater than if the pregnancy were terminated;
	B	the termination is necessary to prevent grave permanent injury to the physical or mental health of the pregnant woman;
	C	the pregnancy has NOT exceeded its 24th week and that the continuance of the pregnancy would involve risk, greater than if the pregnancy were terminated, of injury to the physical or mental health of the pregnant woman;
	D	the pregnancy has NOT exceeded its 24th week and that the continuance of the pregnancy would involve risk, greater than if the pregnancy were terminated, of injury to the physical or mental health of any existing child(ren) of the family of the pregnant woman;
	E	there is a substantial risk that if the child were born it would suffer from such physical or mental abnormalities as to be seriously handicapped.

This certificate of opinion is given before the commencement of the treatment for the termination of pregnancy to which it refers and relates to the circumstances of the pregnant woman's individual case.

Signed ....   **Date** ....

Signed ....   **Date** ....

* Delete as appropriate   D-IDH005329 4-94 C8000 CC38806   Form HSA1 (revised 1991)

Figure 4.2   Abortion certification form (sample).

Health and Safety at Work etc. Act 1974

This Act is of direct relevance to individuals, whether as managers responsible for the safety of staff immediately under their control, or as a member of the team responsible for the health and safety standards in the surgery, hospital outpatient department or clinic. The Health and Safety at Work etc. Act 1974 is a criminal statute and the Health and Safety Executive (HSE) is the enforcement body. Failure to carry out any duty under the Act is an offence and can lead to prosecution.

The aim of the legislation is to provide and create workplace standards for the reduction of known hazards, provision of a safe working environment for employees and adequate training and supervision given as is necessary to ensure, so far as is reasonably practicable, the health and safety at work of employees. All employers must fulfil this obligation. The term 'reasonably practicable' may be inferred from case law and the advice of HSE inspectors.

HSE inspectors have considerable powers, and may enter premises to enforce the law. Although they do not need to ask permission before doing so, they usually telephone to arrange a visit. Sanctions may be imposed upon those who have unlawfully created or permitted hazards, even where no one has suffered an accident or ill health.

Employees themselves are obliged to take reasonable care to help to meet this statutory requirement ('legal duty of care').

Duties of employers and employees

The duties arising from the Health and Safety at Work etc. Act 1974 are not difficult to apply. The legislation requires an employer (including a self-employed person, such as a GP) to provide and maintain a safe working environment, and it establishes powers and penalties to enforce this. The main aim of the Act is to make both employers and employees conscious of the need for safety in all aspects of their work.

Employers' general duties to staff

The most important duty which every employer should fulfil is 'to ensure as far as is reasonably practicable, the health, safety and welfare at work of all his employees' (Health and Safety at Work etc. Act 1974).

Written statement of safety policy

An employer should provide information, training and supervision for staff on health and safety matters. Unless there are fewer than five staff, employers must provide a statement of general policy on health and safety and ensure that it is implemented; employees should be consulted on its form and content. The written statement may be included in your employment contract. However, in a medical practice with fewer than five staff, it is not necessary to give everyone a copy, and the statement can be displayed in a public place.

Safety representatives

Safety representatives are usually appointed if an employer recognises a trade union (e.g. hospitals, health centres). They have a right to challenge the employer on all health and safety matters.

Duties to others using the hospital or surgery

An employer must ensure the safety of anyone using the premises, including patients, medical and pharmaceutical representatives, visitors, builders, tradesmen and health authority staff.

The Act requires the hospital, surgery or clinic to be run so as to ensure that all users of the premises are safe from risks of personal injury, and consideration should be given as to whether there are any potential hazards to elderly or disabled patients.

Notifying accidents and dangerous occurrences

An employer should keep a record of accidents. The HSE should be informed of certain serious accidents that befall anyone using the premises.

Employees' responsibilities

Staff are required to take reasonable care of their own health and safety on the premises, and of the safety of other users of the premises who may be affected by their actions or omissions, and are expected to co-operate with the employer in carrying out these duties. Although employees' duties technically apply while at work, it would be wise to assume that they also apply throughout the time the employees are on the premises (e.g. when preparing coffee or lunch in a staff rest-room).

Staff must not interfere with or misuse any health and safety equipment (e.g. fire exits, fire extinguishers and warning notices).

Health and safety at work – regulations

In January 1993, six new sets of health and safety at work regulations came into force. They apply to almost all types of work activity in hospitals and general practice. Like the health and safety law, they place duties on employers to protect:

- their employees

- others, including members of the public who may be affected by the work being done.

These new regulations are needed to implement six European Community (EC) directives on health and safety at work. At the same time, they are part of the continuing modernisation of UK law, and cover the following:

- health and safety management (revised in 1999)

- work equipment safety (amended in 2002)

- manual handling of loads (amended in 2002)

- workplace conditions (amended in 2002)

- personal protective equipment (amended in 2002)

- display-screen equipment (amended in 2002).

Management of health and safety at work (1999)

The regulations require employers to:

- assess the risk to the health and safety of their employees and anyone else who may be affected by their work in order to identify any necessary preventive and protective measures. Employers with five or more employees should write their risk assessment down

- make arrangements for putting into practice the preventive and protective measures that follow from this risk assessment: they should cover planning, organisation, control, monitoring and review (i.e. the management of health and safety). Again, any employer with five or more employees must put these arrangements in writing

- carry out health surveillance of employees when appropriate

- appoint a competent person (normally an employee) to help to devise and apply the protective steps that the risk assessment shows to be necessary

- set up emergency procedures

- give employees information about health and safety matters

- co-operate on health and safety matters with other employers sharing the same premises (e.g. other health authorities)

- make sure that employees have adequate health and safety training and are sufficiently capable at their job to avoid risk

- give whatever health and safety information temporary staff need to meet their specific needs.

These regulations also:

- place duties on all employees to follow health and safety instructions and report danger

- extend current health and safety laws which require employers to consult employees' safety representatives and provide facilities for them.

Provision and use of work equipment (1998)

These regulations pull together and tidy up various laws governing equipment used at work. These regulations:

- place general duties on all employers

- list minimum requirements for work equipment to deal with selected hazards which apply across all industries and sectors.

Generally speaking, these regulations make explicit what is already provided for elsewhere in current legislation or in good practice. Organisations that have well-chosen and well-maintained equipment need not do any more. The general duties of these regulations require organisations to:

- take into account the working conditions and hazards in the workplace when choosing equipment

- make sure that equipment is suitable for the use intended and that it is properly maintained

- give adequate information, instruction and training.

Manual handling operations (1992)

These regulations replace patchy, old-fashioned and largely ineffective legislation with a modern ergonomic approach to the problems of manual handling. They are important because the incorrect handling of loads may cause injuries, resulting in pain, time off work and even permanent disablement.

They apply to any manual handling operations which may cause injury at work. The manual handling assessment is a specific requirement under this regulation. The safety management regulations include not only lifting loads, but also lowering, pushing, pulling, carrying or moving them, whether by hand or by means of other bodily force. Again, these regulations are supported by general guidance.

There are healthcare areas where staff are at risk in this respect, such as nursing. Employers have to take four key steps.

1   Avoid hazardous manual handling operations when it is reasonably practicable to do so.

2   Assess adequately any hazardous operations that cannot be avoided.

3   Reduce the risk of injury as far as possible, taking into consideration the physical suitability of the employee, clothing/footwear, knowledge and training.

4   Review assessments when changes take place.

Workplace health, safety and welfare (1992)

These regulations tidy up much of the existing legislation, replacing some 35 pieces of old law. They are much easier to understand and make it far clearer what is expected. They cover many aspects of health, safety and welfare in the workplace, setting general requirements in four broad areas:

1   *working environment* – temperature, ventilation, lighting, room dimensions, suitability of workstations

2   *safety* – safe passage of pedestrians and vehicles, windows and sky-lights (safe opening, closing and cleaning), safe materials and marking for transparent doors and partitions, doors, gates and escalators (safety devices), safe doors, gates and escalators, floors, falls from heights and falling objects

3   *facilities* – toilets, washing, eating and changing facilities, clothing storage, seating, rest areas, arrangements for non-smokers and rest facilities

4   *housekeeping* – maintenance of workplace, equipment and facilities, cleanliness, and removal of waste materials.

Following the implementation of the Disability Discrimination Act (1995), the 2002 amendment requires employers to ensure that facilities used or occupied directly by disabled persons at work are organised to take account of such persons.

Employers should ensure that their premises comply with these regulations.

Personal protective equipment (1992)

These regulations set out sound principles for selecting, providing, maintaining and using personal protective equipment (PPE). They are not directly relevant to medical secretaries and receptionists, so further information would be inappropriate here.

Display-screen equipment (DSE) (1992)

Unlike most of the regulations previously listed, the health and safety (display-screen equipment) regulations do not replace old legislation, but cover a new area of work activity. Working with DSE is not generally risky, but it can lead to musculoskeletal problems, eye fatigue and mental stress. Problems of this kind can be overcome by good ergonomic design of equipment, furniture, the working environment and the tasks performed.

The regulations apply to DSE where there is a regular user (i.e. an employee who habitually uses it as a significant part of normal work). They cover equipment used for the display of text, numbers and graphics, regardless of the display process used.

These regulations include the following:

- assessing DSE workstations and reducing risks which are identified

- making sure that workstations satisfy minimum requirements set for the DSE itself – keyboard, desk and chair, working environment and task design and software

- planning DSE work so that there are breaks or changes in activity

- providing information and training for DSE users.

DSE users are entitled to appropriate eye and eyesight tests, and to corrective glasses if they are needed and normal spectacles cannot be used. Again these regulations are supported by detailed guidelines which are contained in the Health and Safety Executive's *Guidance Note on DSE Work*.

The Control of Substances Hazardous to Health Regulations (COSHH) 2002 (amended in 2004)

COSHH regulations set out guidelines for the control of hazardous substances to employers, who have an obligation to protect people exposed to such substances.

The regulations include virtually all substances which are hazardous to health, and clearly set out the essential measures which employers, the self-employed, and sometimes employees, have to take. Failure to comply constitutes an offence under the Health and Safety at Work etc. Act 1974. Substances hazardous to health include those labelled as:

- dangerous
- toxic
- harmful
- irritant
- corrosive
- biological agents
- carcinogens
- asthmagens.

The regulations give guidelines to employers which are based upon principles of occupational hygiene, the key duties being:

- to identify substances hazardous to health in the workplace
- to assess formally (in writing) the risk to employees from these materials
- to control adequately and monitor the risk
- to provide health surveillance where appropriate
- to provide adequate information, instruction and training.

Other less dangerous substances covered by the regulations include disinfectants, clinical wastes and cleaning materials.

GPs, health authorities and other healthcare employers should consider how COSHH applies to the working environment and to their employees, for example:

- the risk from biocides and sterilising agents
- the risk of staff contracting infection from biological samples and waste
- policies and specific procedures are necessary for cleaning medical equipment, and safe disposal of drugs, contaminated needles, dressings and appliances
- staff vaccination status should be reviewed.

Summary of legal aspects

This section has attempted to give an overview of the many and diverse legal aspects involving the work of medical secretaries and receptionists.

On a more personal note, information has been given to provide a basic knowledge and understanding of the legislation that influences the duties and rights of employees and employers working in organisations, large or small.

Useful websites

www.chre.org.ukj
www.gmc-uk.org
www.nmc-uk.org

5

Health and safety in a clinical environment

Introduction

General principles of health and safety at work have already been discussed in some detail. On a practical level, how does this affect the secretary and receptionist working in a clinical environment?

The Health and Safety at Work etc. Act 1974 requires:

- *that any 'plant' in the workplace is safe* – the term 'plant' covers equipment in the work environment, including heaters, sterilisers, electric kettles, plugs and examination couches. Potential hazards include someone getting a shock from an electric kettle due to a plug being incorrectly fitted, or a patient being injured because an examination couch collapses. Occurrences such as these could lead to a charge of having unsafe plant on the premises and ensuing liability. Electrical and mechanical equipment needs to be serviced at least annually

- *that systems of work are safe* – it is important that day-to-day work systems are safe and do not lead to injury. Safe systems normally refer to policy and procedures (e.g. manual handling risk assessment and the use of gloves while handling specimens)

- *that premises are safe* – this includes floors which are uneven and/or slippery or dangerous when wet, outside steps which are uneven and/or unlit at night, and ceilings in danger of collapse, which could all be regarded as unsafe.

First aid at work

Regulations require employers to make adequate provision for their employees in case of injury or if they should become unwell at work. It is advisable, but not mandatory, to have a qualified first aider, although a doctor or a nurse could become an 'appointed person' – but there must be an appointed person available at all times. This person is to take charge of the situation should a serious injury or illness occur in the workplace and is responsible for the first-aid equipment. An 'appointed person', if not fully trained, should have attended a short course in first aid lasting a minimum of four hours, which should include the following:

• resuscitation

• control of bleeding

• treatment of the unconscious casualty.

Following the amendment made to the First Aid Regulations in 2002, any first-aid room must be easily accessible to stretchers, and clearly signposted.

Hazardous substances in the workplace

Control of Substances Hazardous to Health (COSHH) regulations have already been mentioned. Receptionists and secretaries should be aware of hazards arising from the handling, transport, storage and disposal of hazardous substances. Control measures must be in place to ensure that their place of work is not in breach of the law.

The Hazardous Waste Regulations 2004 define hazardous waste as those substances having one or more properties that are hazardous to health or to the environment, as documented in the *European Waste Catalogue*. New regulations came into force in July 2005 setting out new regulations designed to give greater protection to both employers and employees from hazardous waste, and guidelines for its disposal.

Clinical waste

Clinical waste is waste arising from medical practice that may provide a hazard or give offence unless it is rendered safe and inoffensive. Such waste includes human or animal tissue or excretions, drugs and medicinal products, swabs, dressings, instruments or similar substances and materials.

All staff involved in areas where clinical waste arises should be given instruction in waste handling, segregation, storage and disposal procedures and, where appropriate, the use of protective clothing.

Waste segregation

This is achieved by the use of readily identifiable colour-coded containers or plastic bags:

- *black* – normal household waste **only**
- *yellow* – clinical waste for incineration.

There are different categories of waste and different procedures for each category. These include the following:

- soiled surgical dressings, swabs and other contaminated waste from consulting rooms and treatment areas
- syringes, needles, cartridges and glass ampoules ('sharps'). It is dangerous to dispose of 'sharps' in yellow bags, as this is a potential cause of needlestick injuries
- laboratory waste in medical practice, including blood samples, vomit or sputum
- solid-dose medicinal products, small-volume injectables, vaccine and sera*
- urine and other samples containing body fluid.

Secretaries and receptionists will be given appropriate instructions for disposal if necessary. However, the following guidelines should be understood by all those working in medical practice.

Storage of clinical waste

Waste bags must be kept secure from unauthorised persons and entry by animals whilst awaiting collection. They must never be left outside where children may play, or where drug addicts may find used syringes and needles.

*All controlled drugs covered by the Misuse of Drugs Act require special procedures before they can be destroyed. Unused drugs are usually returned to the pharmacy for safe disposal.

Removal of clinical waste

This is arranged on a local basis. Health authorities/health boards will advise on the availability of a collection service. Organisations providing this will arrange to supply services and arrange collection and incineration.

Specimens

Handling specimens

Receptionists in general practice may find that patients leave various specimens on the reception counter unwrapped. It is the receptionist's duty to protect herself and colleagues from potential infection by handling these specimens correctly. For example, either ask the patient to place the specimen in a plastic bag, or use a pair of disposable gloves to handle the specimen. The same system could be used for handling used medicine containers, dressings, tissues, hearing aids, etc.

Transport of specimens

Specimens to be sent to the pathology laboratory by the local collection service must be clearly labelled and accompanied by pathology request forms. Specimens to be sent by post must be packaged in a rigid container with absorbent packing and sent by first-class letter post. The address of the sender should be clearly written on the outside of the package so that the post office can contact the sender if the package is damaged, in order to ascertain the risk to the handler. Specimens sent through the post must be clearly labelled 'Pathological Specimen – Handle with Care'.

The NHS National Patient Safety Agency (NPSA)

The NPSA was set up to tackle and improve the safety of patients in the NHS by learning from patient safety incidents and service failure in the NHS. It collects and analyses information from local NHS organisations, staff, patients and carers, and initiates preventive measures so that the whole service can learn from each case. As well as ensuring that incidents are reported, the NPSA aims to promote an open and fair culture across the health service.

National Patient Safety Agency

Improving patient safety

In complex healthcare systems, things will and do go wrong, no matter how dedicated and professional the staff. And when things go wrong, patients are at risk of harm.

At the National Patient Safety Agency (NPSA) we believe that tackling patient safety in the NHS collectively and in a systematic way can have a positive impact on the care and efficiency of NHS organisations.

The NPSA helps the NHS learn from things that go wrong and develops solutions to prevent harm in the future. We do this by working with patients and staff locally and nationally to foster a culture where errors can be investigated and innovative solutions developed. We also do this by using the results from the collecting and analysing of information from staff and patients via our national reporting and learning system and other sources.

From 1 April 2005, the NPSA's work also includes safety aspects of hospital design, cleanliness and food. This responsibility has been transferred from NHS Estates. The NPSA is also ensuring research is carried out safely, through its responsibility for the Central Office for Research Ethics Committee (COREC), and is supporting local organisations in addressing their concerns about the performance of individual doctors and dentists, through its responsibility for the National Clinical Assessment Service (NCAS). It also manages the contracts with the three confidential enquiries. This responsibility has been transferred from the National Institute for Clinical Excellence (NICE).

We are also working with NHS staff and organisations to promote an open and fair culture, and to encourage staff to inform their local organisations when things go wrong. Working in partnership, the NPSA will help the NHS to establish safety as its first priority.

Visit our website at www.npsa.nhs.uk to learn more about the NPSA and view the tools and resources available to support you in improving patient safety in your organisation.

Figure 5.1   The NHS National Patient Safety Agency (NPSA).

Hepatitis and AIDS

Receptionists are at risk in situations where blood, semen and other body fluids of an infected person can enter the body (e.g. through an open cut). All scratches, cuts and grazes must be covered with a waterproof dressing.

When body fluid has to be mopped up, disposable plastic or latex gloves, a disposable plastic apron and paper tissues must be used *whether or not* infection is present. After use, these items must be placed in a clinical waste collection unit for incineration. Clothing may be cleaned by washing on a hot cycle. Hard surfaces and floors can be wiped/washed with a freshly prepared 10% bleach solution. Skin that has been in contact should be washed with soap and water. Mouth-to-mouth resuscitation should be carried out with a mouthpiece if one is available. Common-sense measures and good hygiene are the best ways to prevent infection.

The likelihood of staff being infected with hepatitis is considerably higher than with AIDS, as the virus survives at room temperature for a much longer duration. Hepatitis B vaccination is available to staff for protection.

Fire Precautions Act 1971

This is the Act that covers fire regulations. However, in medical practices with less than 20 employees there is no need for a fire certificate. Larger organisations (e.g. hospitals and health centres) will have regular fire drills. The local fire officer will check the provision of fire alarms, extinguishers and hoses, and that fire exits are not obstructed and signs are readily visible. The provision of emergency light supplies is also checked.

Medical practices should have their own plans and clearly defined procedures to be followed in the event of a fire. Basic guidelines would include the following:

- *prevention* – check for hazards and try to prevent a fire from occurring

- *fire alert/warning* – who will raise the alarm and dial 999? Who will evacuate the surgery? What is the system for ensuring that everyone in the building knows about the fire? How can more patients be prevented from entering?

- *evacuation* – procedures for evacuating the building. Marshall all staff and patients to one assembly point. Check that no one is missing

- *security* – people are most important. Leave behind all valuables except the appointment book, which will tell you if anyone is missing. This should be taken to the assembly point

- *informing staff and the public* – a notice should be displayed telling people what to do in the event of a fire. The notice should indicate the assembly point and the action to be taken in the event of a fire.

Clinical risk management

Although risk management is not new, its application to clinical medicine is a relatively new concept in the UK. It is a response to increasing medical litigation but, in addition to reducing the chance (or cost) of litigation, it should lead to improved patient care. In a hospital, one of the greatest areas of risk in financial terms arises from patient treatment. Clinical risk management programmes require the active involvement of senior and junior medical staff, nurses and other healthcare professionals. Clinical risk management may be categorised as follows:

- accident prevention

- damage limitation.

Accident prevention means taking steps to avoid adverse outcomes, and it includes the following:

- continuing medical education

- clinical audit

- protocols and guidelines for treatment

- the application of results from previous claims.

For example, a primary prevention step may be for a new member of staff in Accident and Emergency to know which facilities are immediately available and how and when to summon more experienced assistance.

Damage limitation measures either help in the investigation of a problem, or are steps taken to ensure that events or incidents are routinely investigated.

Clinical risk management is not about gathering information and form filling, but rather it is concerned with identifying and analysing the risk and then controlling it. Controlling the risk is the most important element, as the ultimate aim is accident prevention.

Coping with aggression and violence

Violence against NHS staff is becoming more and more of a problem. It requires action at the highest level to find a solution. The Government has promoted a campaign of zero tolerance, which aims to:

- ensure that the public are aware that violence against NHS staff is unacceptable

- reassure NHS staff that acts of violence and intimidation against them are not acceptable, and that action has been taken to combat them.

In 1998, the Government set the NHS targets of cutting acts of violence against staff. NHS trusts published strategies to achieve these targets and to monitor their outcomes.

A requirement of the Crime and Disorder Act of 1998 is that the police and local authorities should work with organisations, including NHS trusts and health organisations, to bring in strategies to combat crime and disorder.

Abuse threat to NHS staff

A survey commissioned by the Healthcare Commission showed that in the past year (2004–2005) 27% of NHS staff had been harassed or abused by patients. This figure rose to 37% if attacks by colleagues were included. In total, 14% of staff admitted to being physically attacked. These figures show that there has been no improvement in the level of threat to NHS staff, despite the policy of zero tolerance.

The NHS Security Management Service (NHS SMS)

In December 2003 NHS SMS launched the strategy 'Protect Your NHS: a Professional Approach to Managing Security in the NHS'. The SMS Legal Protection Unit has successfully taken action against its first offenders and published a range of guidelines to help health bodies to protect their staff and property, and the first wave of new security management specialists is in place locally across the health service.

A significant development in NHS security management is the introduction of local security management specialists (LSMS). Each health body is required to nominate an LSMS who will become an accredited professional and undergo a four-week training programme. The role of the LSMS will draw together many different aspects of security management, starting with their highest priority, namely tackling violence against NHS staff.

Further new measures are planned and it is important that all incidents of violence, abuse, theft, vandalism or other breaches of security are recorded accurately and promptly according to the reporting systems that are in place. Vigilance and co-operation on the part of receptionists and secretaries will ultimately lead to the best possible protection for patients, staff, professionals and property across the NHS. Their role will help to achieve this aim, and they will also be the beneficiaries of increased security in the health service.

Dealing with aggressive callers

Receptionists and secretaries working in the field of healthcare face a number of patients and callers who are potentially violent (e.g. the mentally disturbed, the emotionally upset, or those who are suffering from the effects of drugs or alcohol).

Your organisation will no doubt have a policy for dealing with potentially violent patients. If so, it is up to you to ensure that you know what it is and what you should do. Remember that most of the patients attending your hospital or your surgery are seeking understanding, help and advice about problems which are causing them a certain amount of anxiety. They may become frustrated and aggrieved as they wait for their appointments.

As a patient becomes more upset, this can lead to aggression and the receptionist or secretary may be the focus of the latter. Always deal as quickly as possible with any patient who becomes agitated, especially if they seem to be under the influence of drugs or alcohol. Make sure that you alert the doctor or nurse to the problem as soon as possible.

If a confrontation is developing, try to defuse the situation by talking to the patient in a calm manner, and attempt to reduce their agitation. You may be able to distract the patient from their particular grievance and cool the situation.

You should be on guard to protect yourself from physical attack. If you are trying to appear relaxed and natural you may, for example, put your hands in your pockets – this will leave you defenceless to a blow. If possible, always put a physical barrier (e.g. a computer or desk) between yourself and the aggressor. Discreetly try to attract the attention of another member of staff if it seems as if the situation is going to erupt. If you have a buzzer 'alert' or panic button system, have a prearranged signal and use it.

NHS organisations are installing closed-circuit television (CCTV), which will often act as a deterrent.

Note: The best way to defend yourself from attack is to get out of the way as quickly as possible.

Coping with a personal attack

A personal attack is unlikely to occur, and if you take common-sense precautions you can reduce the risk. Unfortunately, some attacks do occur and you should give some thought to what you would do if you were a victim.

Always remember that personal safety should come before property. Is it worth being injured for the sake of a prescription or some tablets? The police would prefer you uninjured and in a position to give them an accurate description of the attacker.

It is worth considering what you would be prepared to do in self-defence should you be attacked. If other people are nearby, then you must shout to attract their attention. Only you can decide whether to fight back. A woman has the right to defensive action using reasonable force in the case of an attack – for example, by kicking, scratching or by the use of items which are accepted as normally being carried, such as:

• hair-spray

• bunch of keys

• umbrella

• personal attack alarm.

However, it must be pointed out that legally you may not carry offensive weapons.

If you are sexually assaulted or raped, it is important that you contact the police immediately – both for your own sake and for the safety of others. Always bear in mind:

• however difficult or unpleasant the thought, resist the urge to wash or change your clothing – you could be removing important evidence

• do not drink alcohol or take any drugs that might prevent you from giving a clear account of what has happened

• try to remember as much as possible about your attacker.

The police will deal with you with care, understanding and complete confidentiality.

General security and safety in the surgery or hospital

• Challenge all suspicious individuals.

• Do not be taken in by so-called workmen or officials; if they are genuine, they will not mind having their identity checked.

- Keep all valuables and prescription pads out of sight.

- Ensure that petty cash is secured in a locked tin, and kept inside a locked drawer.

- Ensure that consulting and treatment rooms are locked when not in use.

- If you have an identity badge, always wear it.

- Equipment should be security marked.

- Always keep your valuables with you, or lock them away.

Travelling to and from work or whenever you are out and about

You should always be alert to potential danger when travelling by car, public transport or on foot. Remember the following points.

- Think ahead. Get into a safe routine and always use it.

- Avoid walking home late at night.

- Walk purposefully. Do *not* accept lifts.

- When travelling by car, do not give lifts to strangers.

- On public transport, sit near the guard, driver or other women passengers.

- Only use a reputable taxi-cab firm. Ask the cab company for the driver's name and call sign.

- In the event of your car breaking down, while you are waiting for help make sure that you keep the doors and windows locked and sit in the passenger seat so that you do not appear to be alone.

- Avoid using multi-storey car parks if possible.

- Carry a torch with you if you are travelling after dark.

Safety at the end of a surgery or clinic session

Always check that the premises are secure before you leave, and look outside to make sure that no one is lurking. If you see someone prowling or hanging around, stay inside and let someone know. If necessary, contact the police. If you are usually collected by car, wait until it arrives before going out. If you are travelling by public transport and are alone, do not leave so early that you have to wait a long time for the bus or train.

Finally, your local crime prevention officer attached to your nearest police station will be willing to talk to you and your colleagues about coping with aggression and violence, and give practical help and advice to women about their personal safety.

Summary

Health and safety in a clinical environment involves everyone working in the NHS, and medical secretaries, receptionists and all other administrative personnel should work together as a team to promote good practice.

Health and safety is a very complex area which requires commitment from everyone in the health service to aim for the highest standards in all areas. Health trusts must exercise a duty of care to ensure that waste disposal is properly managed, in order to ensure the safety of employees and others.

A survey published by the Healthcare Commission in April 2005 highlighted public concern about hospital cleanliness and the increase in hospital-acquired infections. It is reported that England has the highest MRSA (methicillin-resistant *Staphylococcus aureus*) rates in Europe.

The new *Matron's Charter: an action plan for cleaner hopsitals* charged all NHS staff with the responsibility for controlling infection rates. The target of reducing MRSA by 50% between 2005 and 2008 has demonstrated a determination to address the problem. One of the initiatives that aims to combat the rise in infection rates is the NPSA's 'Clean Your Hands' campaign.

Useful websites

www.npsa.nhs.uk/cleanyourhands
A Matron's Charter: an action plan for cleaner hopsitals; www.dh.gov.uk

6

Practical reception skills in general practice

Introduction

Every receptionist is gifted in some way, for example in dealing kindly with people, having patience, a pleasant speaking voice, etc. In addition to these natural gifts, everyone can acquire skills to help them to do their job better. The most important skill areas are those of communication and organisation, which are covered in other areas of this text. However, there are some skills which are unique to a receptionist in general practice.

All approaches to the receptionist are by patients, or their relatives, who believe that they have a need. They cannot see 'behind the scenes' in the surgery or have any real understanding of the pressures on doctors and receptionists. Receptionists must always bear in mind the perceived need of the patient, no matter how insignificant it may seem from the surgery perspective. Patients are concerned about either their own state of health or that of a family member. It is very important, therefore, that the skills of recognising how patients are feeling and dealing sensitively with them are used constantly. Non-verbal communication and related issues are covered in Chapter 2.

The person responsible for controlling the flow of patients into a number of doctors consulting at the same time needs to have a good system, to concentrate and to remain alert. If other members are fully co-operative in matters such as ensuring that the appointments book or surgery lists are clearly written, or appropriately 'marking off' a patient as arriving, or having been sent into the doctor, then the task is made simpler. However, the person controlling the surgery flow tends to be the one to whom everyone turns with queries. Where are Mrs A's results? Where are the notes for child B? Do I need to do a claim form for child health surveillance? How many extras are there? When will Dr C be free to see the rep? And so on. If telephone answering is also part of the picture, it can be very difficult to keep on top of who is where, and what needs to be dealt with next.

Smooth surgery flow is made easier if the preparation for surgeries has been carried out properly. Where an appointment system is used, it is sensible to take out all the medical records well before the start of surgery, and check that all of the test results and hospital letters relating to these records have been filed. It can also help the practice finances if stickers are used on the records to indicate that smears are due or pill forms need to be signed, which the receptionist can then act upon by drawing the doctor's attention with a note, or completing a claim ready for signature.

As patients leave the consulting-room, follow-up appointments need to be arranged and appropriate advice given about requirements for some health promotion clinics (e.g. to bring a urine sample). Maintaining neat work areas during consulting times makes tidying at the end of surgery considerably easier. However, even if it is not possible to keep tidy at the busiest times, it is important that quieter times are used to the full to return working areas to order, file medical records, and check that doctors' rooms have been tidied and that stocks of disposables topped up.

Telephone answering can be an especially difficult task for the doctor's receptionist. Any incoming call may be about a patient who is bleeding, appearing to have a heart attack, or experiencing some other medical crisis with a child. Therefore the procedure for dealing with emergencies must be clear and the telephone must never be left to ring for an indefinite period. The telephone must be answered in preference to dealing with a patient standing at the reception desk. However, it is also essential that any patient at the desk is acknowledged with a smile, so that they know they will be dealt with when you are free.

The receptionist is also required to be a fount of all knowledge. For example, the following can be helpful in finding and giving out appropriate information efficiently:

- keeping telephone directories of often used numbers, or hospital internal directories, along with other service information sources

- a list of subjects of leaflets kept available for patients in the waiting-room and brief notes on developments in trends in health promotion

- a list giving addresses and telephone numbers of self-help groups and voluntary organisations

- awareness of changes to surgeries and clinics, and changes in local hospital, community and social services.

It is especially important that the receptionist knows the limits of her own authority (i.e. when and to whom to refer for advice).

The receptionist is also responsible for keeping an eye on the waiting-area to:

- make sure that the patients who are obviously unwell are not troubled by unduly active children

- generally keep a watchful eye on the waiting-area, and note if any patients appear to be unduly distressed or extremely unwell

- maintain a pleasant ambience by ensuring adequate ventilation or heat

- tidy the waiting-area of toys, magazines and leaflets at the end of each surgery or clinic.

Thankfully, it will rarely be necessary to clean up whilst patients are waiting (e.g. if a patient is literally sick in the waiting-area or treads something unpleasant-smelling from the pavement into the surgery!).

Keeping the doctors happy is yet another set of tasks for the receptionist. Most of the time this will entail keeping the surgery flow steady, not allowing too many interruptions in consultations, providing tea or coffee at the right times, and making sure that records, results, letters and other essentials are all available when required. Not too much to ask!

Individually controlling surgery flow, answering the telephone, dealing with patients at the desk, and keeping the doctor happy are not too difficult to achieve as separate items, but in the real world of the reception office there is rarely the opportunity to concentrate on one task at a time. The skill is in being able to readjust priorities constantly, without forgetting the ones that slip to the bottom of the mental pile.

Dividing up the duties so that, for instance, one person controls surgery flow, another concentrates on answering the telephone, and another does repeat prescriptions and perhaps deals with queries, can go some way towards reducing the pressure. However, it is also impossible to adhere rigidly to such a plan. It is essential that receptionists work in a team, not only keeping on top of what they are supposed to be doing, but also having their eyes open to see when a colleague needs help, and being able to adjust their own priorities to step into the breach.

Various tools, such as log books, message books, having good systems in place, having clear procedures for dealing with routine issues, and knowing whom to turn to with queries, all help. However, the ability to juggle ten priorities at one time is both an art and a gift. Being self-controlled, planning work, and being as efficient about it as possible means that anyone with a degree of intelligence, who wants to, can achieve a certain degree of competency. However, there will always be some people who enjoy this kind of pressure (only feeling the strain sometimes) and some to whom it is a strain all the time.

First impressions

First impressions count. A receptionist will often be the patient's initial point of contact with the organisation, and they will make assumptions (positive or negative) about the treatment that they are likely to receive from that first point.

Record keeping and general administration

In any business it is essential to keep records. For example, where a receptionist may be delegated the task of keeping control of stocks of forms and stationery, or petty cash, it is essential that adequate documentation is maintained. Alternatively, a receptionist is likely to pass messages to a variety of people in the course of a working day. Keeping a record of messages ensures that not only does the right message get passed, but the person who took the message, the person who received it, and when, can all be substantiated.

Written communication

Although technology is moving on apace, there is still the need for handwritten communication – messages and notes from one person to another. It is obvious that any handwritten communication should be legible, but often in haste it is easy to forget this, and to fail to ensure that any other person can read a scrawled message, entry in an appointment book or list of names, etc.

Messages

Some offices have preprinted message forms which prompt message takers to collect all of the necessary information as they go. Another option is to use a message book with columns drawn up, so that it is easy to check whether a message has been received. It is important not only that there should be adequate systems for communicating messages, but also that responsibility is taken to ensure that the systems work properly.

Message-boards

Dry-wipe white-boards are extremely useful for putting up short-term reminders and messages, provided that one person is delegated responsibility for wiping off messages as soon as they become redundant!

Letters and memos

Receptionists may be required to send out letters and memos. As a general rule these are likely to be routine (standard) documents, where a master copy is used to generate photocopies, into which names and addresses, dates and data can be inserted by hand. However, technology has made it possible for receptionists with little or no formal training in secretarial or wordprocessing skills to generate printed letters from the computer. It is vital to remember that the image of the practice/hospital is presented via written communication, and therefore it is vital that presentation standards are met. There are conventions about letter layout (e.g. whether commas are used at the end of every line in an address or how many spaces are left between the end of a letter and 'Yours sincerely'). Where training is not given in these details, a poor impression will be conveyed to anyone who expects normal conventions to be observed. Therefore the setting of practice standards is a valuable guide to ensure that everyone produces written communication to the same standard.

Practice newsletters

Most doctors' surgeries and GP practices now produce a quarterly newsletter (usually available at the reception desk) that informs patients of any recent developments and changes which may have taken place. It may, for example, include information about the following:

- new clinic sessions
- changes to appointments systems
- new repeat prescription procedures
- staff changes – the arrival of new healthcare professionals, receptionists or other administrative personnel, etc.

Practice newsletters may also provide information about hospital waiting times, influenza vaccination clinics and other topics of interest to patients or their relatives.

Organisation

Systems and organisation are essential to the smooth running of a reception area. Some people are blessed with a natural ability to be organised. Those who are not need to apply far more self-discipline in order to initiate and maintain systems. Everyone needs to know what is expected of whom, using what, and by when.

Similarly, individuals need to be organised in their use of time. The receptionist who retains control of the tasks to be completed avoids personal stress. Too much stress will inevitably lead to mistakes, poor handling of patients, and a general deterioration in standards of service.

Box 6.1

Take time out to:

1   make a list of the tasks you perform every day, every week, and once a month:

- make a week plan

- block off the times on the week plan when you have no option but to be 'demand driven' (e.g. on reception desk for a busy surgery/clinic)

- fit other tasks around these blocks at the optimum time

2   make a 'to do' list

- break down large items into small stages

- realistically allocate items from your 'to do' list into your working week

3   discuss your findings with your supervisor so that any queries regarding priorities can be resolved to their satisfaction.

Using the simple example of stocks of forms, unless there is a system for ensuring that stocks are maintained, there is every likelihood that either one day stores will run out, or that scarce storage space will be taken up by unnecessarily large supplies.

Since there are many supplies needed, it is helpful if a system is set up and maintained with the same degree of commitment from everyone.

Initial skill is needed to think through the best and simplest way of organising any particular aspect of reception. After that, discipline and commitment from all team members are essential to maintain the system.

Maintaining the office and reception areas

In order to ensure the comfort and well-being of patients, relatives and other visitors, an effort needs to be made to keep the public areas tidy and smart. This must be a priority, because untidiness can be a hazard and gives a general impression of sloppiness.

Ensure that:

- the area is kept tidy and free from hazards. Some visitors are likely to have visual or physical disabilities

- hazards are reported promptly and immediate action is taken to minimise the danger

- fire exits are clearly indicated and kept unobstructed

- notices and information leaflets are kept up to date, and are clearly and neatly displayed

- an up-to-date supply of magazines, etc. is available for visitors to read.

Mail

Mail should be correctly sorted and date stamped on receipt. Any enclosures should be securely attached and missing items reported promptly. The mail should then be passed to the appropriate person for action.

When sending out mail, check that names and addresses are correct and clearly legible. Envelopes and parcels should be securely sealed. All of the mail you deal with should be handled promptly, as it relates to patients' health and any delay could be dangerous.

If you are suspicious of any mail received, local security arrangements should be followed. Check with your manager if you are unfamiliar with these.

It is appreciated that, for example, in some medical practices the receptionist or secretary may not be involved in handling or dealing with mail.

Stock control

The purpose of a stock control system is to keep track of such items as stationery, computer hardware, drugs, dressings, linen, sundry equipment, etc. that the practice owns. A stock control system is necessary to avoid two pitfalls:

1 *having too much stock* – money that is tied up in stock cannot be used for any other purpose, and if the stock is perishable or becomes obsolete as time passes, it may be difficult to recover this money in full

2 *having too little stock* – if essential items are scarce, patients may face long delays or inconvenience.

The ideal situation, and the one that a good stock control system aims to produce, is to have adequate stock on hand – neither too much nor too little.

Stock control also acts as a deterrent to wastage and pilfering. A good system will show when losses are occurring, and the knowledge of this may deter pilferers. It should also highlight the points at which losses are likely to occur from other causes.

Records of stock levels are obviously essential to any large-scale control system. The records may be on index cards, or a computerised stock control system may be in operation. Goods are stored until they are needed, and are released by the storekeeper only when he or she is presented with a duly authorised document, such as a requisition note.

Petty cash

Small amounts of expenditure for goods or services are usually paid for out of petty cash since the amounts are too small to be paid by cheque (e.g. stamps, milk bills, small stationery items). Secretarial or clerical staff may be responsible for controlling petty cash, and the system most commonly used is known as the *imprest* system.

The imprest amount is drawn from the account each week or month, through the main cash-book. The sum is estimated to cover all small expenses throughout the agreed period, and is referred to as the 'imprest' or 'float'. The petty cash is kept in a locked cash-box. During the month, payments are made from the imprest, and all expenditure must be covered by a petty cash voucher or a receipt. The voucher should be signed by the person receiving the money. The vouchers and receipts should be numbered and filed for purposes of audit.

A separate petty cash-book is maintained which analyses the expenditure, and at the end of the month a sum of money is drawn by cheque to restore the amount of the imprest to the original sum.

Helping to maintain a safe environment

Health and safety at work legislation is intended to safeguard all employees, patients and visitors to the workplace. Individual employees are required to ensure that they do not endanger their own health or safety, or that of their colleagues, patients or visitors. Potentially dangerous situations and unknown or potentially hazardous substances must be treated with the utmost care.

The legislation is detailed and complex. At the minimum, all staff must ensure that:

- there are no trailing wires
- filing-cabinet drawers are kept closed
- chairs and other obstacles do not block walkways or fire escapes
- fire extinguishers and exits are clearly indicated
- any known hazards are marked clearly and problems reported to the appropriate manager
- visitors are informed of any known hazards
- potentially violent situations are defused as far as is possible

- care is taken when handling specimens, especially with regard to spillages, and hands are washed after undertaking this task.

Coping with aggression and violence

Communication is often the key when dealing with conflict of this kind. Good communication can play a vital part in defusing potentially difficult situations or avoiding them altogether, but equally, poor communication can increase levels of frustration and anger which then erupt in violence (*see* Chapter 5). We have to consider carefully what messages our words and movements are conveying. Are they contradictory? We can tell when someone is saying one thing but means something quite different. Perhaps it is someone we know well, and we can therefore judge their statements on the basis of what we know of them, but it is equally likely that they are strangers, and the truth is conveyed by their stance, facial movements, etc. (*see* Chapter 2).

Procedures manuals

Many organisations are using Standard Operating Procedures (SOPs) as part of the implementation of BS5750 (British Standards Institution is the world's leading standards organisation and facilitates the setting standards, inspections and quality, which is accepted internationally. BS5750 is the world's most popular management system and was introduced to help organisations build quality into the way they work). These SOPs state who does what, how they should do it, and how often, etc.

Within reception offices there may not be the need to have SOPs for every activity or task, but a manual of key procedures may be helpful. The administrative processes of stock control and petty cash are two examples which should be documented in a specific procedure. The procedure document may be just one side of A4 paper with the vital information summarised in a table, but it should include details of who is responsible, what steps are taken, how frequently, and any special notes. Filing these procedure sheets into a looseleaf folder allows additional procedures to be added or existing procedures to be updated whenever necessary. Apart from encouraging a uniform approach to performing tasks, these written procedures form a useful resource, especially for new staff who may have been told how to do something, but have forgotten or need to clarify the details.

Information technology (IT)

Practices still vary enormously in their modes of working, size, number of staff, equipment available, and capability of using their technology.

Computers

Where a practice has the patient database on computer, the advantages include:

- logging and generation of repeat prescriptions

- checking registration status

- checking smears, and other screening status

- checking health promotion data

- receiving email

- making appointments

- checking immunisation data and records, etc.

- receiving information from hospitals, health authorities and trusts.

If this is linked into an appointments system, the difficulties of manual appointment books (e.g. illegible writing, pages messy with cancellations, two people not being able to use the book at the same time, handwritten surgery lists for pulling out records) are all circumvented.

The major disadvantage is when the system 'goes down'. All of this increased efficiency then disappears, and returning to manual methods, no matter how temporarily, results in unavoidable delays and disruption.

Reference is made to IT for written communication in Chapter 10. Suffice it to say here that staff who could only ever write letters are now able to use wordprocessing to generate mailmerged letters, or to produce their own letters to patients with very little training. Spreadsheets can be used either to collect data (for display in tables, graphs and pie charts) or to present doctor and staff rotas.

Desktop publishing software can be used to generate leaflets, posters and handouts. Technology saves time for some tasks, while for others it does not save time, but it does make it possible to produce professional-looking documents (e.g. rota charts, posters).

For those who enjoy using the computer, it is essential that the latter does not become an obstacle between the patient and the receptionist. It is as rude to continue to type away absorbed by the machine as it is to continue to talk to a colleague or take a telephone call without acknowledging the presence of a patient.

The advantages of technology to receptionists include:

- ease of presenting professional standard documents, and speed of finding, generating and transmitting information

- efficiency in dealing with issues.

The major disadvantages to receptionists include:

* reliance on the electronics, so that if the computer 'goes down', everything has to go on hold
* the danger of losing the personal touch.

Fax

The fax machine has the following important uses in general practice:

* return of urgent blood results
* notification of discharge from maternity wards
* passing on complex information
* making claims to health authorities/health boards with regard to patient registration, etc.

Electronic mailing systems have now almost completely replaced the transmission of information by fax.

The Internet

The Internet is a world-wide system of information technology networks, providing a global, on-line computer network that connects governments, universities, organisations and many other networks and users. The service provides:

* access to information
* on-line conversations
* information exchange
* conferences
* electronic mail.

It also has the ability to access remote computers and send and retrieve files. It began in 1984 and is now estimated to have over 50 million users, with an estimated one million new users joining each month.

Electronic mail

Electronic mail (email) is a telecommunications system that enables the users of a computer network to send messages to other users throughout

Figure 6.1 The basic structure of an electronic mail system. A message is sent via a telephone line and stored in a central computer. The message remains there until the recipient calls up the central computer and collects the message.

the world. Telephone wires are necessary to send the signals from terminal to terminal. Email subscribers may send messages by computer by 'dropping' the communication into a central computer's memory bank by means of a modem. The recipient 'collects' the communication by means of an individual password and access-logging to safeguard against unauthorised user access to the system. Figure 6.1 shows the basic structure of an electronic mail system.

Although many GPs still continue to request investigations on pathology request forms, with results sent back to the practice on paper, email is increasingly being used by GPs to receive electronically the results of pathological tests initiated by the practice. The way in which electronic results are used will depend on both the procedures and protocols within the practice and the features of the GP system linking with the hospital laboratory. The main benefits of laboratory links include:

- a significant reduction in the need for GPs or administrative staff to telephone the laboratory for results
- releasing administrative staff time through not having to type in test results
- the patients are impressed!

Photocopying

The photocopier is a great time saver. However, lack of training in office standards and procedures can result in poor-quality work and failure to maintain the equipment properly. Good-quality originals are essential for producing fine-quality copies. A ring binder can be kept near to the photocopier with photocopy originals in clear plastic wallets. (Yellow highlighter pen does not show up on photocopies, so use one to write 'original' to ensure that the original is easily identifiable and does not get circulated by mistake.)

The scanning, storing and printing of documents electronically have in many cases removed the need to photocopy documents, reports, etc.

The effect of technology on staff is to make their lives a lot easier in some ways, and to make aspects of work available to them for personal development. The disadvantage for people who are afraid of technology is that they may get left behind and their value falls because they cannot take an equal share in routine workloads.

A receptionist is now required to have a wide range of skills. Apart from dealing with people on the telephone and face to face, retrieving and filing medical records and filing away letters and reports, the receptionist generally needs to have keyboard skills and a willingness to learn how to use the latest technology.

Appointment systems in general practice

The role that the medical receptionist plays is crucial to the successful running of an appointment system. Nearly every patient who sees the doctor makes his or her first contact through the receptionist. The receptionist channels patients into the appointment system and runs the system once the surgery has started.

The receptionist has to calm the agitated patient, explain and cope with doctors' absences on emergencies, and translate unstreamed demand into a rational framework.

It is important to run an appointment system as effectively as possible, for both the doctor's and the patient's sake – even a few dissatisfied patients can very quickly lead to an unhappy practice. A well-run system reflects the general efficiency of the practice, and puts less strain on GPs and their receptionists.

An efficient appointment system should benefit both doctor and patient. Benefits to doctors include:

* effective organisation of workload

* more efficient management of time

* it limits the number of patients seen in one session

* patients' records are left on doctors' desks in advance of the surgery session

* less waiting-room space is required

* the duration of the consultation can be varied according to predetermined need.

Benefits to patients include:

- being able to plan their day

- they should not have to wait a long time to see the doctor

- there are fewer people in the waiting-room, so less likelihood of cross-infection.

The perfect appointment system is neither so rigid that it excludes emergencies, nor so chaotic that it keeps those who have made appointments waiting for an excessive length of time. The number of patients booked for each surgery session should bear a close relationship to the speed at which the doctor works.

Patient dissatisfaction arises from being unable to get an appointment without delay. Appointment systems should therefore be flexible to allow those patients with urgent problems to see their doctor very quickly.

'Urgent' and 'emergency' are both subjective and emotive terms, and perhaps receptionists should be encouraged to delete them from their vocabulary! They could be replaced with 'will it wait until tomorrow?'. However, your practice will have its own procedures for dealing with such requests from patients.

Types of appointment system

Times of booking for patients can be arranged in various ways, and each practice or doctor will decide which system suits them best.

Whatever system is used, it is essential for the frequency of appointments to match the doctor's consultation rate, and for sufficient time to be left for patients who need to be seen and fitted in at short notice.

Your surgery may use one or a combination of the following types of booking:

- sequential booking

- block-release booking

- limited block booking.

All of these systems have the flexibility for patients to be seen quickly if necessary. There are several ways to deal with 'extras' to be seen despite a full appointments book:

- they can be fitted in between booked appointments

- provision can be made for patients with urgent problems to be seen after the booked surgery

- one doctor in the practice, on a rotating basis, can act as 'mopper-up' and see the extras instead of carrying out a booked surgery

- block-release booking allows 'holes' to be left in the appointments book which cannot be filled until the beginning of the day on which they are entered.

Electronic appointments

Appointments both to see the general practitioner and to see the nurse, phlebotomist, etc. are in many medical practices made by the receptionist using the computer. This allows speedy access to all booked appointments and highlights any free spaces which may be available. Hard copies can be printed off as a back-up, but doctors and nurses have access to computers and can check their own booked patients.

In addition, in some authorities it is possible to make an appointment directly for a patient consultation with a consultant at the local hospital by linking straight into their system.

Whichever method your practice uses, it is essential that the receptionist knows exactly what to do.

Follow-up after missed appointments

Patients who fail to keep their appointments for cervical cytology and immunisations will either be sent a letter or telephoned with a further appointment. If patients do not attend, doctors may not achieve their targets for cervical cytology and child immunisation.

The medical records of non-attendees for routine appointments may be marked 'DNA' or 'did not attend', and this information may also be entered on the practice computer. However, this procedure may vary according to practice protocol.

If the doctor has given the patient advice about follow-up appointments, tests, etc., it is important to check their understanding of the instructions given. They may need to be given a letter or an appointment card with the details of their next appointment. If a patient seems to be confused about what has been said, it is doubly important to encourage them to wait and have a word with the doctor or nurse before they leave. The patient may need to be directed to the correct place for any tests which are necessary. After the appointment, the notes will go to the secretary for any letters that are needed.

Many practices are now using a fully computerised appointments system to provide a more effective method of making appointments for their patients, and to replace the appointments book which can only be used by one receptionist at a time. A major benefit to the practice is that appointments can be made by as many reception staff as there are terminals.

Medical records

A medical record is the history of a patient's treatment as an outpatient, inpatient or both. The record is vital because it provides a means of communication between doctors, nurses and other members of the care team about investigations, diagnosis, observations, treatment prescribed and progress. It acts as a reminder, and can be used as an educational instrument for trainees, for research, for informing medical negligence cases and other legal purposes, and for gathering statistics such as those that are needed for planning future services.

Records contain much confidential information, and all those with access to them have a legal responsibility to maintain confidentiality. Computerised records present a particular challenge to confidentiality. This is examined in more detail in Chapter 7.

Two Acts of Parliament allow individuals access to their medical information. The Access to Medical Reports Act 1988 gives an individual in England, Wales or Scotland the right to see medical reports prepared for insurance or employment purposes. The Access to Personal Files and Medical Reports Order 1991 for Northern Ireland affords similar rights there. The Access to Health Records Act 1990, which applies in England, Wales and Scotland, establishes an individual's right of access to their own medical records. In certain circumstances, access can be granted to other individuals. The Act also provides for the correction of inaccurate information. Access can be refused in certain cases if, in the opinion of the record holder, disclosure would cause serious harm to the patient (*see* Chapter 4).

Medical records were standardised when the NHS began to provide some uniformity between hospitals, although some local variation still exists.

In the UK, the medical records held by general practitioners are unique: they follow patients throughout their lives from the cradle to the grave. Medical records show patients' names, demographic details, and information about previous illnesses and significant episodes in the lives of their subjects, unlike hospital records, which often only cover a specific episode of hospital attendance (e.g. for appendectomy or hysterectomy).

The purpose of the medical record

The basic function of the medical record can best be described as an *aide-mémoire*.

- It gives a method of recording events in a person's life. It traces from birth the record of a patient's illnesses, treatments, investigations and other significant events.

- It is a channel of communication. The GP writes in the medical record, giving details of his or her findings, treatment and diagnosis of a patient's condition. This becomes a permanent record and communicates that information to those individuals who have the right of access (e.g. another partner in the practice, the practice nurse), or to another doctor at a later date.

- It acts as a record of outside health contacts. When the patient attends a hospital outpatient department, or has an investigation, information is provided, and if it is correctly filled in, the patient's record contributes to the total knowledge about the patient.

- It provides a record of all treatment and all of the drugs given during a patient's lifetime.

- It is a medico-legal record. If a medical or legal problem arises at any time, the patient's medical records will be required to support any action taken.

Box 6.2 The four main functions of medical records

1   A permanent record of significant events

2   A medico-legal record

3   A file for hospital and laboratory reports and letters

4   An aide-mémoire

Thus it is vital that medical records are kept securely and the information contained therein is stored in an orderly, systematic way. This can be achieved by:

- ensuring that all of the continuation sheets are arranged in chronological order, hopefully starting from birth, and fixing them in a permanent way (e.g. with a treasury tag), so that new continuation cards can be easily added

- keeping hospital records, copies of GPs' letters and any other correspondence in chronological order and fastened together

- dealing with the results of any investigations in the same way

- keeping a summary sheet on which the major and significant diseases or allergies are entered. This should be kept in the front of the medical record envelope (MRE)

- keeping prescription summary cards, which are also useful as a permanent, easily seen record of all drugs prescribed

There are many other forms of record card that can be used for specific purposes, such as the child immunisation card, repeat prescription summary, obstetric record, contraceptive record, etc.

Medical receptionists and secretaries should not discard anything from a medical record envelope without the doctor's permission.

Storage of medical records

There are different ways of grouping medical records and different types of records. The most commonly used record is the small-size medical record envelope (7 × 5.5 inches) or the A4-size folder.

Some practices separate male and female records, but the majority file them together. There may be occasions when families are filed together in an A4 family folder. Every practice has its own system, but there are three main methods of storage:

1   *lateral* shelving, where records are placed side by side on shelves in alphabetical order, with alphabetical guides
2   *vertical* filing in multi-drawer cabinets, which should have alphabetical guides on the outside of the drawers
3   *carousel* or rotary filing cabinets.

A tracer or marker card should always be inserted whenever a file is pulled, and removed once the medical record is back in place. The receptionist or secretary should always check to see whether a new continuation sheet is required for doctors to record their findings.

Whatever system of filing is used in the practice, accurate filing is essential. It should be possible to pull and refile records quickly and accurately.

Electronic records

In April 2005, the National Programme for Information Technology (NPIT) became part of an agency of the Department of Health called NHS Connecting for Health, which is delivering the NPIT. It has also taken on some of the functions of the NHS Information Authority, which has been disbanded.

Over the next ten years the NPIT aims to connect England's 30 000 or so GPs to its 300 hospitals and thereby enable patients to access their personal health and care information. Information will be quickly transferred, including healthcare records, appointment details and prescription information. Up-to-date research will be accessible to both healthcare professionals and patients when it is needed. This programme will also support patient choice (*see also* Chapter 10).

NHS Care Records Service

The NHS Care Records Service will connect GPs and NHS trusts in a single national system, providing all NHS patients in England with an individual complete medical record that gives details of all key healthcare treatments in the health service or social care services. All doctors, nurses and other healthcare professionals with a legitimate need for access will be able to view patient information 24 hours a day, seven days a week. The first phase was completed in 2005 and includes the following:

- booking of outpatient appointments

- viewing of patient information by healthcare professionals.

It is anticipated that the final phase of the project will be completed in 2010. Please refer to Chapter 10 for further information.

Primary Care Information Service (PRIMIS)

PRIMIS gives free help to primary care organisations to enable them to make the best use of their clinical computer systems. Information facilitators are funded locally, and through PRIMIS they give GP practices training in information management skills, recording data and analysing data quality. PRIMIS also provides a comparative analysis service focused on key clinical issues, giving feedback and interpretation of results, and in addition it offers support in developing action plans to improve data quality. NPIT is currently procuring a new service that will build on the success of PRIMIS (*see also* Chapter 10).

Confidentiality of medical records

The medical record itself has a statement at the bottom saying that it is the property of the Department of Health. However, the protection of the contents for purposes of confidentiality is the responsibility of the doctor and practice staff. Secretaries and receptionists must adhere to the rules of the practice established by the doctor with regard to who may access the information contained in the records.

Practice staff must never divulge any information contained in medical records, and great care must be taken to ensure their safe custody. Remember that many people call into the practice and may be able to see over the reception counter and read things upside down. Cleaners and maintenance staff may come into the practice when letters and other confidential information have been left lying around.

There are certain legal issues pertaining to access to medical records and data protection. These are explained fully in Chapter 4.

Much information about patients, their medical history, investigations, prescribing records, etc., is now stored on computer, but the principles of confidentiality still apply.

The medical record and information systems in general practice

The medical record is an important part of the overall information system for general practice. The record serves the needs of:

- preventive medicine
- at-risk groups of patients
- quality control measures – patient recall, performance review
- practice planning – administration and finance
- education – doctors, staff, trainees and patients
- research.

The age–sex register

The practice population can be well served by an age–sex register, which may be either a manual system or computerised, to help to identify patients at risk.

It can be used for:

- meeting targets
- screening 'at-risk' patients and chronic disease groups
- an age–sex register of the practice population.

Disease or diagnostic index

Once again the system of identification of patients who have certain diseases may be either maintained manually or stored as computer data. In its simplest form in a manual system, the notes can be colour-tagged according to the system established by the Royal College of General Practitioners, which has identified eight disease groups. For example:

- red – sensitivities
- brown – diabetes
- yellow – epilepsy
- green – tuberculosis
- blue – hypertension
- white – long-term maintenance therapy
- black – attempted suicide
- black and white chequered – measles.

The presence of a coloured tag means that the disorder is or has been present. However, the absence of a tag can never imply the absence of such a disorder.

Summary

Information technology is influencing and changing many of the systems that have been used in general practice for many years. This is a time of great change, and receptionists and secretaries may feel threatened by the pace at which technology is advancing. Many practices are striving to achieve a 'paperless' practice, and patients' medical records are already being stored in computer systems.

Advances in information technology are rapidly changing the face of general practice. Many changes have been introduced since the last edition of this book was published, but the next few years will see many more ways in which GP practices are organised. It will be an exciting, challenging, yet rewarding time for all of the staff involved in the electronic NHS.

7

The hospital service

The patient's route through the hospital

The process begins with a visit by the patient either to their GP, or to an Accident and Emergency (A&E) department, or to one of the few direct-access services offered by some hospitals (e.g. walk-in clinics for genitourinary medicine). A GP visit results in a referral, leading to an outpatient appointment, a place on a waiting-list, attendance at a pre-assessment clinic and then admission. A direct visit to the hospital may result in a waiting-list place or even immediate admission, with the GP being informed afterwards. Alternatively, a GP refers the patient via electronic booking for day surgery (e.g. hernia repair), assesses the patient using the hospital protocol, and then books them directly on to the hospital day-surgery list. Otherwise, in some hospitals a system is in place whereby at the time of the outpatient appointment an admission date is agreed between the patient and the consultant, a pre-assessment is carried out at the clinic and the patient is admitted to hospital. This excludes the period of uncertainty while the patient is on a 'waiting-list'. Once in the hospital, the patient may be treated as an inpatient or as a day case, with access as necessary to diagnostic services, operating theatres or treatment departments.

On discharge, a summary of treatment given and follow-up needed is given to the patient's GP. Community support may be arranged, and follow-up clinic appointments may take place either in the GP's surgery or back at the hospital itself, before the patient is fully discharged (*see* Figure 7.1).

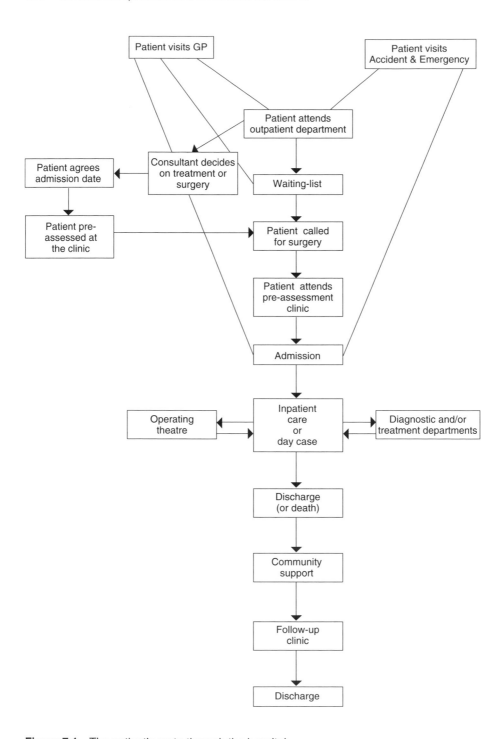

Figure 7.1   The patient's route through the hospital.

Outpatient appointments

A referral letter or specially designed referral form is sent by the GP to the appropriate consultant with an outline of the patient's condition. In exceptional circumstances a telephone referral can be made. The consultant decides how urgent the case is, and when the patient should be seen. A letter or form is then sent to the patient with details of the appointment.

If a patient has failed to turn up for a hospital appointment, this is drawn to the attention of the consultant, who decides whether another appointment should be sent or whether the GP should be informed first.

Outpatient appointments may be made centrally, or in each department, or in a mixture of both. In many hospitals the system is computerised. Each consultant generally decides how appointments are made (whether in blocks or singly), the amount of time allocated to each patient, and how many new patients and how many follow-up patients are to be booked in each clinic. New pilot systems in which patients are being given a confirmed admission date at the time of their consultation have shown that fewer patients are non-attenders, thus resulting in more efficient use of theatre time.

Referrals need not always be from a GP, but can be from the hospital's own A&E department, from another clinic, transferred from another consultant during or after treatment, or from another hospital.

On-line booking

An on-line appointment booking system has been piloted which enables GPs to book patients directly into specific consultant clinics. The 'RAPPORT' (rapid access project program for outpatient review and treatment) system enhances existing appointment booking systems. It provides a 'seamless' link between the hospital and general practitioners via the GP 'LINKS' system, giving direct access to outpatient clinics and day-case clinics.

Using the RAPPORT system, patients who do not necessarily need to see a consultant (e.g. for a hernia repair) may be booked directly by their GP for surgery, with full details of the GP's examination being mailed to the consultant (see Chapter 10 on using information technology).

Electronic booking (Choose and Book) will underpin the Government's policy of enabling patients to choose which hospital to attend at a date and time that will suit them. The implementation on a national basis was completed and replaces the 'RAPPORT' system.

Preparing for clinics

When preparing for a clinic, the first task is to ensure that the patient's notes are ready for doctors to refer to during the consultation. The importance of this cannot be overemphasised, since missing or incomplete notes will result in serious difficulties for the doctor and delays for the patient. It is sensible to allow as much time as possible.

Clinic lists will be available from the appointment book or computerised patient administration system, showing all those due to attend. Case notes are then retrieved or 'pulled', double-checking for the right patient using not only their name but also their date of birth and hospital or NHS number. Checks are made that results of tests and other investigations, X-rays, etc., which were ordered after the previous visit are available.

Receiving patients

When a visitor arrives at reception you should go through the following stages.

- Smile and greet them courteously.

- Establish their identity and the reason for their visit.

- If the visitor has arrived at the wrong clinic in a busy hospital, give them clear and accurate directions and, wherever possible, provide them with an escort. This is particularly important if they are confused or distressed.

- If the visitor is a patient booked into the clinic, ask them to take a seat and explain to them:

  – which doctor will see them
  – how long they are likely to have to wait
  – where they can obtain refreshments
  – where the toilet is situated.

- Deal patiently and cheerfully with any queries the patient may have, and if you cannot answer their questions yourself, find someone (e.g. a nurse) who can.

- If there is likely to be any delay in the patient being seen, try to find out how long this is expected to be, and give the patient a diplomatic and apologetic explanation.

- If the patient has language difficulties, obtain an interpreter or linkworker.

You should always be aware that the visitor may be experiencing discomfort or may be worried about the visit. This should be taken into account in all dealings with patients, their relatives and friends.

Admissions from the waiting-list

Admissions from the waiting-list (elective admissions) are usually handled by an admissions office, which is also responsible for keeping an accurate bed state for the entire hospital. Beds are not occupied at all times, although the hospital will try to maintain occupancy to the maximum in order to make best use of resources. Elective admissions will fill a proportion of beds, but there must be the space and flexibility to be able to accommodate unforeseen demands. A pattern will have emerged over time, and the hospital will plan the use of its beds accordingly.

Admissions on to wards for day-case treatment, day surgery, or for the delivery of babies may be booked directly by those departments. Lists of expected admissions are given to each ward daily and copied to the records department so that case notes are made available.

The NHS Improvement Plan set a target maximum waiting time of 18 weeks between referral and first outpatient appointment, to be achieved by December 2008. Patients will have the right to choose from any provider that meets the Healthcare Commission's standards within the price that the NHS will pay. All patients who have to wait longer than six months for an operation are already offered the option of an alternative place of treatment.

Accident and Emergency admissions

When a patient is brought into A&E by ambulance, the drivers will pass on whatever information they have obtained, and the receptionist will check what previous records exist for that patient. Treatment will not be delayed for this information if it is urgently needed. Specific procedures are followed if the patient is a road traffic accident victim, where ambulance transport costs are recovered, usually from the driver's insurance. Special arrangements also exist for suspected non-accidental injury of a child.

Every hospital has its own procedure for major accidents, and will rehearse it in conjunction with the emergency services from time to time.

Follow-up after admission

When a patient is discharged from hospital, the medical staff prepare a form for the patient to hand to their GP. A form is also completed for financial purposes, showing the diagnosis and any operations performed. After discharge, a full summary is sent to the GP.

Not all patients leave the hospital alive. Following the death of a patient, the relatives must of course be dealt with in a kind and sensitive manner.

Home from hospital support

An increasing number of hospitals are finding that a patient can be discharged more successfully if they are offered support at home for a period of time following their return. Home from hospital teams consist of trained nurses and care support staff who arrange to visit frequently and regularly over a specified period to help the patient to adjust to being back at home. Help is offered with a range of activities designed to increase the patient's confidence in being able to cope at home. A speedier and more successful discharge both helps the patient and keeps acute hospital beds available for those who need acute nursing care.

Day cases and ward attendees

More and more people opt for surgery as a day case where this is possible. Strict criteria apply, and not all procedures or all patients can be dealt with in this way. Every effort is made to ensure that the patient has someone to collect them at the end of the day. An overnight stay will always be available should the patient's condition require it.

Most hospitals have taken steps to increase the proportion of work done on a day-case basis but, interestingly, the assumption frequently made by patients that this is a cheaper option for the NHS is not often borne out. Many hospitals find that variable costs for tests, disposables, etc., are higher per patient, and since they will be putting more patients through each bed (one per day rather than, for example, one per two or three days), total costs for these items can escalate. Staff costs can be higher because of the greater dependency of each patient, and the fixed costs associated with the building are not reduced until there has been a major shift from inpatients to day cases, allowing ward closures and large staff reductions.

The hospital team

Hospital staff fall into a number of professional groups, as described below.

Medical staff

- *Consultants* are responsible for the diagnosis and treatment of patients referred to them.

- *Junior doctors in training*, house officers, senior house officers and specialist registrars, work for a consultant's firm. Although they are qualified doctors, they are in training for specialist roles.

- *Other doctors*, such as staff grades, clinical assistants, hospital practitioners and associate specialists, are also attached to a consultant's firm. They are below consultant grade but are no longer in training.

Nursing staff

- *Modern Matrons* have been appointed to be responsible for 'cleaning up' hospitals and so reducing the number of patient-acquired infections. Community matrons will be appointed by 2007. The aim is to help the NHS to achieve its target of reducing emergency hospital admissions by 5% by 2008.

- *Nurses and midwives* provide the regular care for patients as set out in the care plan, and administer drugs and treatment under the direction of the doctor. Psychiatric nurses work to ensure patients' mental health. Midwives care for mothers and babies and have special status as independent practitioners, which allows them in certain circumstances to practise without a doctor's prior instruction.

- *Clinical nurse specialists* offer an alternative way to access primary care by running nurse-led clinics. Many diagnostic tests that were formerly performed in hospital will now be performed by nurses, GPs or others with specialist interests.

- *Healthcare assistants* and nursing assistants work with qualified nurses and therapists to deliver non-technical care to patients.

- *Nurse consultants* have a specialist knowledge and qualification that equip them with the skills necessary to advise on patient treatment and care.

- *Nurse prescribers* have the konwledge and training to enable them to write prescriptions for certain drugs (*see* Chapter 11).

- *Nurse practitioners* are nurses with specific training to allow them to practise independently, in some cases taking on responsibilities that are usually held by junior doctors. They may run clinics, assess priorities in A&E departments (known as triage), and undertake some treatments.

New contract for consultants

In 2003 a new consultant contract was agreed which aims to provide a more effective system of planning and timetabling consultants' time, duties and activities with regard to the NHS. It is designed to meet local service needs and priorities. For consultants, it means greater transparency about the commitments that are expected of them.

Existing consultants were given the choice of whether or not to take up the new contract, but newly appointed consultants are only offered the new contract.

Therapy staff

- *Physiotherapists* diagnose and treat patients' difficulties with movement and rehabilitation after illness or injury, using exercises, manipulation and a range of equipment.

- *Occupational therapists* help patients to resume a normal life through activity-based treatments and the provision of aids to living, such as special tools and appliances.

- *Dietitians* advise patients and other care staff on the best food and drink for particular conditions. They also advise on intravenous and other drip-feeding procedures.

- *Speech and language therapists* help patients with communication difficulties, especially after a stroke or other injury to the head, throat or chest. They also treat children who have communication difficulties.

- *Hearing therapists* assist patients with hearing difficulties and support those with hearing aids.

- *Pharmacists* provide specialist advice on appropriate drug treatments, including drug interactions, and supply drugs to inpatients and outpatients.

Diagnostic staff

- *Pathology staff* carry out a range of tests which are grouped into categories. Haematology staff perform tests on blood. Cytology staff study the nature of cells (especially cancerous or other diseased ones). Histology staff study tissues to detect disease. Microbiology staff test urine, faeces and other body fluids for parasites and bacteria. Virology staff look for the presence of viruses. Chemistry staff look for the presence of chemicals which may cause illness or be a symptom of disease.

- *Radiography staff* take X-rays for interpretation by a radiologist. They perform various treatments, such as barium meals or dye injections, to show up particular parts of the body. They also use ultrasound to examine babies in the womb, and to detect disease (e.g. a tumour) in other parts of the body. Computed axial tomography (CAT) scanning uses a computer to reconstruct an image of a layer of tissue in the body. Nuclear magnetic resonance imaging (NMRI) uses radio frequency radiation and a magnetic field to produce anatomical sections of the body.

- *ECG staff* use an electrocardiograph to take readings which describe the functioning of a patient's heart, for cardiologists to interpret.

- *EEG staff* use an electroencephalograph to produce a picture of brain activity, by placing small electrodes on the patient's head to measure electrical impulses. Consultants in EEG interpret the pictures.

Support workers

- *Non-clinical support departments* include chaplaincy, catering, cleaning, porters, security, building, engineering, linen and laundry, and transport.

Management and administration

- *Management departments* include the chief executive's team, general managers, directors of nursing and midwifery, business managers, human resources, finance, payroll, information and marketing. Management departments are also responsible for clinical audit and non-clinical audit and governance, complaints and legal services.

- *Administrative support* is provided by admissions, registry and medical records.

Clinical audit

The term 'clinical audit' embraces the audit activity of all healthcare professionals, including nurses, doctors and other healthcare staff. It is a widely used tool within hospitals, and is defined as the systematic and critical analysis of the quality of clinical care, including the procedures used for diagnosis, treatment and care, the associated resources and the resulting outcome and quality of life for the patient.

As a general principle, audit should be professionally led and should focus on improving outcomes. It will have the greatest impact if it forms part of routine clinical care. It should be seen as an educational process and be an important part of quality programmes. It must respect confidentiality at the individual patient or clinician level, and take into consideration the views of the patient and their carers.

Star ratings

The Healthcare Commission has been responsible for reviewing every trust's performance and awarding an annual performance rating, usually referred to as a 'star rating'. Star ratings do not always reflect the local issues, which may themselves affect the rating.

A new performance framework for the NHS and social care came into effect in April 2005. It sets out the quality that all organisations which provide NHS care, including foundation trusts and those in the private and voluntary sectors, will be expected to meet or aspire to.

The Healthcare Commission has devised a new system for assessing the performance of NHS organisations from 2005, based on the core and developmental standards framework. It will examine the following two areas:

- *getting the basics right* – core standards, national targets, financial position and management, value for money, and findings from other regulatory bodies

- *making and sustaining progress* – the four national priorities set out in the Department of Health's Public Service Agreement, namely to improve the health of the population, to improve the health of people with long-term conditions, to improve access to services, and to improve the patient and user experience.

The new system will replace the existing star ratings, which were published for the last time in July 2005.

What is a medical record?

A medical record is the history of a patient's treatment as an outpatient or inpatient, or both, at a particular hospital. If it is known that a patient has attended another hospital, a copy of that treatment record should be included in the current hospital medical record. A complete record prevents duplication and facilitates future care. In most cases, at present, the most complete medical records are the GP's notes, as they follow patients when they move around geographically. GP records should also contain details of any hospital treatment received by the patient, as well as any letters and summaries from hospitals which the patient may have attended.

Why have medical records in hospitals?

- They are of most value in the treatment of patients, as a reminder and as a means of communication to doctors, nurses, etc. of what has been given and with what effect, and investigations which have been made and the results.

- They are an educational instrument and, as such, are used to teach medical students, nurses and other students.

- They are used for research.

Storage of medical records

Every hospital has its own system, but there are three main methods:

- lateral filing systems – files are arranged side by side on shelves
- vertical filing systems – files are stored in multi-drawer cabinets
- rotary (carousel) systems.

Each of these methods has its advantages and disadvantages. The security of any area in which medical records are held is of prime importance.

Case notes

Although medical records were standardised when the NHS was instituted in order to ensure uniformity of record-keeping procedures, these vary from one hospital to another. A hospital receptionist or medical secretary who moves from one hospital to another is unlikely to find herself handling exactly the same procedures. Standardisation overall does exist but without rigidity.

Case notes basically follow the same pattern everywhere, being contained in A4-sized folders and consisting of five sections:

- identification
- medical
- nursing
- correspondence
- results (e.g. pathology tests, X-rays).

Identification section

This section allows space for the following information:

- hospital's name and code number, which is usually printed
- patient's name, address, status and telephone number
- patient's postcode
- patient's date of birth
- GP information
- consultant
- hospital number
- patient's occupation
- patient's religion
- NHS number
- next-of-kin information.

Medical section

This section is for doctors' use only, and generally consists of the following:

- history of present complaint
- past medical history (PMH)

- family history
- patient complains of (PCO)
- on examination (OE)
- differential diagnosis
- investigations
- treatment.

Nursing section

This section contains the observations of nursing staff (recorded only when patients are admitted):

- nursing record
- temperature, pulse, respiration (TPR) – graphic records on special sheets; also used for blood pressure, micturition and bowel function
- intake and output charts (record of all fluids taken orally or by transfusion and excreted).

Correspondence section

This section will usually include the following:

- GP's referral letter or pro forma referral
- consultant's reports to GP
- letters to and from other consultants or professionals.

Other information

The records may also contain the following:

- prescription charge
- social history
- theatre/surgical operation sheet
- consent form
- anaesthetic form.

The order of all these sheets inside the folder will vary from one hospital to another, and ideally the order is printed either on the front or inside the cover. Each section of the case notes is generally filed in chronological order.

Master index

In theory, each patient should have only one medical record. This rule is broken by the law which states that the records of patients who attend the genitourinary clinics must be kept separate from any other medical records belonging to such patients. Psychiatric medical records of patients are also usually kept separately, with just a note placed in the main medical record stating where and when the patient attended for psychiatric care. In order to reduce the number of patients with several medical records, a master index is kept.

The master index is an alphabetical list of patients who have attended the hospital. It can be kept on cards and filed manually, on microfiche, on computer, on microfilm or on optical disc. The information recorded is usually basic, consisting of surname, forename(s), sex, date of birth, home address, marital status, sometimes the date of first attendance and consultants seen, religion, date of death and patient index number.

The master index record for the A&E and emergency eye departments usually consists of alphabetically filed cards of attendees there.

Filing room/medical records library

This is the hub of the medical records department. It is often located on a lower-ground or ground floor because of the weight of all the records. Security in this area is of prime importance. Unauthorised access cannot be allowed.

Within the library, files will be organised according to a strict system. A number of different filing systems exist as follows, although in most hospitals medical records are filed by patient master index number. Colour coding is often used to prevent misfiling.

Master index number – terminal digit (12 34 **56**)

Six numbers are required. 12 34 **56** gives 56 as the terminal digit, 34 as the middle digit and 12 as the first digit. Divide the main area into 100 sections, 00 to 99, and these divisions give the foundation for terminal digit filing. This means that 56 will be in main section 56. The main sections are again divided into another 00 to 99 subsections, so 56 will be placed in subsection 34 and 12 will be placed behind 11 and before 13 in subsection 34. Although this may sound complicated, with a little practice it is easy to work and helps to reduce misfiling.

Middle digit (12 **34** 56)

A similar process to terminal digit is followed, but the numbers are followed in a different order:

- straight numerical (1, 2, 3, etc.)

- date of birth – alphabetical

- surname – alphabetical.

Medical records procedures for departments

Accident and Emergency records

If a patient arrives in hospital by emergency ambulance, the drivers will fill in the ambulance book stating what information they have collected about the patient. A receptionist will check if there are previous A&E records and/or medical records, and will obtain them as quickly as possible. Treatment does not wait until these are found. If there is no record of previous attendance, an A&E record is started with what information is available. This may be difficult if the patient is unconscious and unaccompanied, so there must be a follow-up should the patient eventually go on to a ward. Nurses usually record any property that the patient is carrying, but a receptionist could be asked to do so, with a witness.

If the medical record shows that the patient has current appointments for outpatients, or has been booked for admission or for theatre, these departments must be informed if the patient is not going to attend.

Outpatient records

Outpatients attend the hospital after a letter of referral from their GP. Many GPs use a referral form. This gives basic details of the patient which help to find any existing medical records. The letters go to the consultant or senior registrar of the department concerned, and an appointment is scheduled according to urgency. A list for each clinic is drawn up, and the medical records for all patients booked are then prepared.

A copy of the manual list or the computer list in 'pulling' order is produced ('pulling' is jargon for the actual gathering together of medical records from the filing shelves). Filing-room staff, clinic clerks, receptionists or admission-office staff may do this, and again this will vary according to each hospital's system.

The person preparing for the clinic will receive a copy of the list, and must obtain the medical records and laboratory tests, X-rays, etc. which were ordered at the previous visit. These results must be in the medical records and the X-rays ordered so that they are at the clinic. The medical records are also checked to ensure that there is paper on which the medical staff may write, and are 'stamped' or written up with the date and the consultant of the clinic.

If the patient is new to the hospital, the case notes are partially written up (in order to save paper and time), but the details are not confirmed on the computer until the patient has actually arrived. On arrival, all of the patient details are checked and any missing information is obtained. If a manual system is used, this information is put on the master index card.

Day-case records

These are usually handled by the department or the ward concerned. The medical records department is contacted for the necessary records before the patient arrives, where possible. The procedure is broadly the same as that described above for outpatients.

Maternity records

In many hospitals these records are retained by the woman throughout her pregnancy and only kept by the hospital after her confinement.

Admissions and transfers

A list of expected admissions is sent to each ward daily. A copy of this list is sent to the records library so that the medical records can be on the ward before the patient is admitted. Usually the ward receptionist does the check on the contents of the medical records, as described above for outpatients.

Retention of records

The usual retention periods are as follows:

- *obstetric records* – 25 years, or eight years after the death of the child but not of the mother

- *children and young people* – until the patient's 25th birthday, or 26th if the entry was made when the young person was 17 years of age, or eight years after death if sooner (ten years for GP records)

- *psychiatric patients* (within meaning of Mental Health Act 1983) – 20 years after treatment is no longer considered necessary, or eight years after death (ten years for GP records)

- *all other personal health records* – eight years after the end of treatment (ten years for GP records).

Destruction of medical records

Medical records departments will have a written destruction policy which will have been agreed by both clinical and administrative staff.

Destruction of medical records should only be carried out by authorised personnel in accordance with the written policy, by incineration or shredding. Destruction should be monitored to ensure absolute confidentiality. A record of instruction should be retained.

What's new in medical records?

There is a trend towards permitting patients to carry their own notes. This is particularly useful in cases where patients have a chronic condition such as diabetes or high blood pressure.

For many years, maternity patients have carried a 'co-operation' card which has proved highly successful and parent-held records are more common where young children are concerned.

It has been found that patients do not lose their records, and that being responsible for their own record may even be beneficial. The main disadvantage is that hospital records may not be complete, which could prove difficult in cases of litigation.

'Smart' cards the size of credit cards have existed for a number of years, and trials have been conducted in parts of the UK on their use to carry health records. They have also been used by pharmacies to track prescriptions. However, smart-card systems have not yet been implemented comprehensively in the NHS.

Smart cards contain a large amount of information in a small microchip, but they require sufficient locations with input devices and readers before they can be universally adopted. They are commonly used in France and other European countries for health purposes.

The computer-based electronic record has also been on trial in the UK, but it does not seem likely that electronic records will replace paper records in the foreseeable future.

NHS Care Records Service

A single electronic record system to which all providers of care have access is becoming increasingly necessary as patients attend various organisations at different times. They are treated and/or cared for by different care professionals (e.g. the independent sector, NHS trusts and social services).

The role of the secretary in hospital

The vital link

The secretary's role is a vital one in the smooth running of the department. Frequently the first point of contact, the secretary acts as a representative of those for whom she works, and also represents the whole organisation. She provides a link between members of the healthcare team, and between them and the outside world, and her involvement can ensure that scarce resources, such as a consultant's time or a theatre list, are used as efficiently as possible, and to the very best advantage. Diplomat, oiler of wheels, the one who gets things done, the one who remembers that important detail that everyone else has forgotten – the role is as varied as it is complex.

Core knowledge and skills

All secretarial posts in healthcare services require a body of core knowledge and skills which underpin all activities within the job. These include good interpersonal skills, respect for confidentiality, the ability to use appropriate medical terms, an understanding of the principles of medical ethics and etiquette, and sensitivity to the physical and psychological needs of patients and their carers.

In addition to these, there is a requirement to comply with legal requirements concerning working practices, and to be aware of and work within other health and safety regulations.

The NHS Knowledge and Skills Framework

The core of knowledge and skills for every job in the NHS is now captured within the NHS Knowledge and Skills Framework (KSF) profile. This profile describes the knowledge and skills required for every job, and also the levels of knowledge and skills necessary to progress.

The KSF outline describes six core areas for each job. In addition to these, each job will have its own combination of some of the following.

* Communications –
  processing, distribution and despatch of mail; efficient and courteous use of communications systems, including telephone, answering machines, pagers, fax, telex and electronic mail

* Correspondence –
  identifying, prioritising and responding to correspondence for own action, including letters, circulars, invoices and statements; passing on correspondence for others' attention promptly

* Organising work schedules –
  maintaining diaries, visual planners, computerised and other scheduling aids; making and confirming appointments; planning and prioritising own work schedule; co-ordinating assistance where necessary

* Information –
  using manual and computerised filing systems; responding to requests for and producing information from internal and external sources, including public documents, timetables and statistics; presenting information in different formats

* Office administration –
  managing and controlling office stock, following appropriate ordering procedures; dealing with faulty equipment; maintaining a petty cash system

- Meetings –   preparing and producing agenda
                                papers and minutes; booking rooms,
                                refreshments and audio-visual aids;
                                arranging room layout; attending meetings to
                                take notes, and producing formal records of
                                business undertaken

- Reception –   receiving and screening visitors, and
                                assisting them wherever possible

- Documents and reports –   preparing and producing documents,
                                including reports, tables and statistics;
                                arranging copying, collating and binding

- Appointment systems –   answering requests for and allocating
                                appointments; following booking-in
                                procedures, registration procedures,
                                preparing case notes, paperwork, tests,
                                results, etc. for clinics or surgical lists

- Waiting-lists –   accurately compiling and prioritising
                                waiting-lists (manual or computerised);
                                arranging and confirming appointments,
                                handling queries and undertaking follow-up
                                action as necessary

- Health and safety –   ensuring that the work area is kept free from
                                hazards; recording and reporting accidents
                                and unsafe features; following safe methods
                                for lifting and handling heavy or bulky items;
                                following procedures for raising the alarm or
                                summoning assistance; adhering to
                                procedures for handling specimens

- Patient care and   dealing with patients and carers with
  support –   sensitivity, identifying and responding to
                                their needs; adhering to the requirements of
                                the Patient's Charter; arranging transport and
                                escorts, following procedures for handling
                                patients' property

8

Private medicine

Introduction

Throughout the development of the National Health Service, the private care sector continued to operate and remained a minor element of the total health provision, until the 1980s when it rapidly expanded in response to the various constraints on the NHS. The number of both health insurance schemes and private providers has expanded, and by 1989, 13% of the population in the UK was covered by private medical insurance, and approximately 17% of all inpatients were treated privately and 17% of elective surgery was carried out in the private sector. At the same time there has been an increase in the number of private residential and nursing homes. By 1997, 12 million people were receiving treatment covered by private medical insurance, and this together with GP commissioning and the 'choose and book' system that is now available has resulted in an increased number of private hospitals and clinics.

A number of medical secretaries and receptionists are now employed in private medicine, either working for specialist physicians or surgeons in their consulting rooms, or in a private clinic or hospital.

Although their function is essentially similar to that of secretaries and receptionists working in NHS organisations, there are certain differences in working practice (*see* Chapters 6 and 7).

Changes in the relationship between the NHS and the private sector

The NHS Plan states that 'for years there has been a stand-off between the NHS and private sector providers of healthcare. This has to end'. As a result, the new arrangement is set out as a concordat between the NHS and the private sector, covering private and voluntary providers of healthcare. A national framework for partnership includes a set of guidelines helping primary care groups and trusts when they commission services. A patient would remain an NHS patient even if they were treated in the private sector, and as an NHS patient care would remain free at the point of delivery.

Private clinic or hospital

Patient contact and communication

Receptionists welcome patients on arrival at the clinic or hospital, where they may be asked to complete registration forms. They will then direct them to the appropriate departments, which include the following:

- outpatients
- physiotherapy
- X-ray
- diagnostic imaging
- pathology.

They may take telephone calls from patients, give advice on payment protocol, make an appointment for them to see a consultant or other healthcare professional and, if necessary, refer to a nurse for advice.

Facilities

Private hospitals and clinics provide patients with rooms equipped to the highest standards to ensure a relaxed and comfortable environment, which is conducive to rapid recovery and convalescence. Rooms are generally equipped with *en suite* bathroom facilities, as well as telephone, colour television, videos, and DVD players. Other amenities available will probably include the following:

- library and internet connections
- mail, fax and secretarial services
- counsellor (for patients and their families)
- hairdressing and laundry services

- chiropody

- private ambulances.

Private hospitals offer a wide range of menus, providing the opportunity for patient choice, designed with 'healthy eating' in mind, and providing a nutritionally balanced diet. Light refreshments are usually available for visitors.

Operating theatres and diagnostic and treatment departments are usually equipped to the highest standards and use the latest technology. Resident medical officers provide 24-hour medical cover for patients.

Customer care

Customer care is always an important element in a private clinic. For example, tea or coffee is offered free of charge to patients who are waiting in outpatients.

In an effort to improve the quality of care, receptionists will present questionnaires to patients, who are asked to comment on all aspects of their care through the outpatient department, including reception, nursing, X-ray, phlebotomy, etc.

Other aspects of customer care are the same as would be expected from a similar NHS organisation (e.g. arranging for a wheelchair or porter, and generally helping a patient as is felt necessary).

Changes and developments

The independent acute healthcare sector has seen many changes in recent years. The increasing demands of clinical governance (*see* Chapter 13), the regulation of independent hospitals, the National Frameworks, public expectations and media interest in healthcare have all combined to provide a challenge to management teams in the private sector.

Quality assurance

Private medicine is a highly competitive market, and hospitals and clinics have accordingly developed quality assurance programmes to maintain and improve standards. Regular audits and reviews are held to monitor achievements against written standards. Patients' opinions and views are an integral part of performance audit. Staff training and development are generally included as initiatives contributing to providing expert care and attention to patients at all times.

Healthcare Commission

Private hospitals and clinics are subject to inspections by the Healthcare Commission in the same way as their NHS counterparts, and this plays an important role in regulating the independent healthcare sector through registration, annual inspection and enforcement. The Healthcare Commission also investigates any serious failures in the provision of healthcare.

Telephone skills

In common with other areas of medical practice, the receptionist in a private clinic or hospital deals with all types of people – elderly, vague people, overseas visitors who cannot speak English very well, impatient people and demanding people. Patience, tact, understanding and a good telephone manner are just as essential in a private setting, as well as the ability to deal with situations efficiently and quickly because there is always another call waiting to be dealt with!

Appointments

When patients make appointments, they are asked for the following basic information:

- name – surname and forename(s)
- age, if necessary
- telephone number
- address
- whether they have medical insurance.

An appointment card is sent to the patient with directions on how to reach the clinic, and details of car parking availability. The patient is informed of consultation costs (if known) and the cost of any investigations. Any special instructions that may be necessary will also be sent to patients prior to their appointments.

Outpatient hospital/clinic registration procedure

On arrival at reception, patients are asked to complete a registration form giving the following information:

- name, address and telephone number

- name and address of general practitioner

- name of consultant

- insurance company (if appropriate), membership/registration number and authorisation number of reference

- method of payment; they may be asked to sign to confirm that they are willing to pay for their treatment on the day.

In some private clinics, patients may be encouraged to pay for outpatient treatment on the day of their appointment, and to get any insurance forms signed there and then by the consultant, so that there will be little or no delay in reimbursement.

Inpatient registration

If a patient has to be admitted, a more detailed form is given to them for completion, which also asks for details of their insurance cover.

Patients may be asked to give details of their medical history and/or current medication.

Pathology, X-ray and diagnostic imaging

Receptionists and secretaries may generate accounts for patients who are attending for these outpatient procedures, and in some instances may request payment at the time of investigation. Alternatively, patients may be asked to call at the accounts office to settle their account. The accounts protocol varies between different private organisations.

Medical records

Consultants in a private hospital or clinic will bring patients' notes with them and keep them in their personal possession.

The only records that are kept at the clinic will be screening records such as well-woman, executive screening, breast screening, etc. All records of work generated by the staff are retained at the clinic.

Records of nursing and inpatient procedures are retained by the private hospital or clinic in the same way as in an NHS trust. Patients are allocated a hospital number on admission.

Mail – incoming and outgoing

Mail addressed to doctors is generally kept in pigeon-holes for their collection. All outgoing mail, accounts, letters, etc., are collected by the mail room at the end of the day for posting.

Patient accounts

The preparation and processing of patient accounts is a major part of the receptionist's job. They are prepared on the computer, and may have to be ready for patients when they leave the clinic. Private hospitals and clinics have the facility to collect cash, accept payment by means of credit cards and cheques, and often have a 'Switch' machine.

Systems

All accounts for the day will be sent to a main accounts department for filing. Any outstanding bills can be demonstrated on the computer screen. There is a variety of software available, but a frequently used system is 'Compucare'.

Liaison with other healthcare professionals

Receptionists have regular contact with consultants and their secretaries, as well as with physiotherapy, X-ray and nursing staff at the clinic. They will have frequent telephone contact with almost every sector of the medical field, including laboratory staff, doctors, secretaries, NHS hospitals, clinics (private and NHS), psychologists, etc.

From time to time, they may be asked to contact a patient's private medical insurance company for information about levels of cover, etc.

Waiting-areas and consulting-rooms

Consulting-rooms are checked and maintained by nursing staff, except for stationery items, which are the responsibility of the receptionists.

Doctors will usually liaise by telephone to ask for their patients to be taken to them, and the receptionist or nurse will show them into the doctors' rooms.

Waiting-areas are kept clean and tidy by frequent visits from housekeepers. Catering staff will ensure that there is a supply of tea and coffee and remove dirty cups from the waiting-area. Magazines are always available for patients.

The secretary in private practice

The role of the secretary in private practice is a diverse and varied one that requires qualities and skills in addition to those needed for secretarial duties. In many instances the secretary will be working on her own, apart from the days when her consultant is seeing patients at the practice. This means that decisions of a non-medical nature may have to be made.

Reception and secretarial duties

A great deal of the secretary's time is involved with answering the telephone, dealing with patients' enquiries and making appointments.

Once an appointment has been made for a new patient, a file is made up containing basic patient information and details of private medical insurance cover, in readiness for the initial consultation.

The secretary may be asked by her consultant to organise investigations (pathology, radiological examination, etc.) for patients when necessary, and to arrange for external referrals (e.g. physiotherapy, other consultants). Admission to the hospital or clinic may also be arranged for the patient.

From time to time the secretary will need to liaise with her NHS counterpart, either to leave a message or to contact the consultant when he or she is working in the hospital department.

She will be responsible for keeping the consulting-room, waiting-room and her own office tidy and generally ensuring the comfort of patients while they are waiting to see the doctor.

It is advisable for the secretary to ensure that patients are made aware of the costs involved in private treatment for both self-paying individuals and those with health insurance. Patients who will be undergoing surgery must be informed of the procedure codes and the expected fees for the surgeon, anaesthetist and any others involved. It should also be mentioned that if any additional procedure is performed, it will be reflected in their final account. Insured patients must be advised to contact their company in order to obtain authorisation for the procedure, and to find out whether there is likely to be a shortfall on the fees. This is not within the remit of the secretary, as the policy is between the insurance company and the patient, *not* between the company and the consultant, but the secretary may need to contact the company in a supporting role.

Some insurance companies are now offering direct invoicing and payment through electronic data interchange (EDI). The latter is an established method for sending messages directly from one computer system to another, particularly business transactions. Some insurance companies have set up their own electronic billing systems.

Clerical duties

On a daily basis mail has to be sorted and incoming correspondence attended to as appropriate. Photocopying of insurance or medical reports may be necessary from time to time, and messages sent or received by facsimile (fax) transmission dealt with accordingly. Correspondence will have to be posted and a supply of postage stamps maintained at the practice.

The secretary will usually be responsible for petty cash for purchasing office sundries and maintaining supplies of stationery and other items.

She will pull patients' records prior to consultation and check that the results of investigations previously requested are complete. Following consultation and any further action that has to be taken, the notes will be filed away.

Email messages (both incoming and outgoing) are becoming a popular means of communication. The receptionist or secretary should always check for messages at least twice a day.

On a daily basis, too, all incoming cheques and cash should be checked against the outstanding patient accounts.

Secretarial skills

Good secretarial skills are important, including typing and competent use of word-processing systems. Many consultants prefer to dictate their letters and reports on to a dictating machine, but some still prefer their secretaries to use shorthand. Usually a combination of shorthand and audiotyping skills is desirable.

A knowledge of medical terminology and medical abbreviations is always useful, but not necessarily essential. A good medical dictionary, common sense and an ability to learn the specialist terms will usually suffice.

In private practice, with no nurse in attendance, the secretary may be asked to act as a chaperone during the consultant's examination of the patient.

Practice management

The secretary in private practice will find that, in addition to her other duties, she is also a practice manager. The good manager will update existing systems to ensure that the practice operates effectively and in an efficient way. She will be responsible for sending patient accounts and, if necessary, will remind patients that settlement of their outstanding account is overdue, and will follow up unpaid accounts on a regular basis, as well as patient account reconciliation. Any long-standing overdue accounts will be referred to a debt collection agency when necessary.

At least once a week, all cheques and cash should be entered in the accounts book and paid into the bank. An accounts book should also be kept for recording income and outgoings for office supplies, catering, etc.

The secretary will reconcile the petty cash account on a regular (usually monthly) basis, and will recommend when accounts should be paid by the consultant.

Another financial aspect of the work of the medical secretary in private practice will no doubt be to operate a payroll (perhaps for only one person), to calculate her own PAYE and NI contributions, and to make year end returns to the Inland Revenue. She will also be responsible for ordering any supplies necessary for the doctor's consulting-room and her own office requirements.

In the current climate of admission only a few hours before surgery, it may be necessary for the secretary to form a close liaison with the hospital and anaesthetist and to obtain details of the present medication, medical history and general health of the patient. This would allow appropriate investigations to be pre-booked and performed quickly in the short interval between admission and surgery.

Summary

It will be noted that the role of the receptionist and secretary in private practice is very similar to that of their counterpart working in an NHS organisation, but with greater financial and accounting responsibilities.

An essential quality is to be able to deal with patients in an efficient yet sympathetic manner, and to understand the emotions and concerns experienced by patients when they enter a clinical environment. Although it is desirable for secretaries and receptionists to have a knowledge of medical terminology and other clinical aspects, a competent person will learn these as they carry out their day-to-day duties.

9

Forms, fees and finances in general practice

Introduction

Primary care trusts (PCTs) are the cornerstone of general medical practice. They run primary care services (and also community services) and commission care from a wide range of providers.

The Government has stated that the health service should be 'primary care led' and, reflecting this, PCTs have control over approximately 75% of the NHS budget.

Contracting

General Medical Services contract

The *Red Book* General Medical Services (GMS) contract was a set of statutory arrangements made by the Department of Health between primary care organisations (PCOs) and individual GPs. The new GMS contract is a UK-wide contract. However, at a local level the practice-based contract is individual to each practice, but is derived from the regulations based on the standard GMS contract. The practice-based contract between the PCO and the practice will need to deal with such matters as the range of services to be provided, the quality of care and the practice's resources. The statutory arrangements governing the old GMS contract ended on 31 March 2004.

The new contract allows GPs greater flexibility with regard to the services that they offer. It has enabled some doctors to reduce their workload, while others have taken on new services, and remuneration is adjusted accordingly. Some practices may choose to hand over responsibility for evening, weekend and bank holiday services to their local PCT, which must ensure that the same level of services continues to be provided.

GP practices must provide *essential* services (i.e. treating the sick, terminally ill patients and patients suffering from chronic disease), but they are able to opt out of providing *additional* services, such as the following:

- child immunisation

- child health surveillance

- maternity services

- contraceptive services

- cervical screening.

It would appear that most practices are maintaining or expanding the services that they provide.

Enhanced services

These are essential or additional services delivered to a higher specified standard (e.g. extended minor surgery). They may also be services that are not provided through essential or additional services. They may be specialised services undertaken by GPs or nurses with special interests or by allied health professionals, or they may be services that address specific local health needs.

Direct enhanced services (DES)

These are enhanced services that PCOs must commission. These services are classified and include the following:

- services to violent patients

- influenza immunisation

- minor surgery

- childhood vaccinations and immunisations.

National enhanced services (NES)

These services have minimum specifications. General practitioner involvement in NES is voluntary. These services include the following:

- intrauterine contraceptive device fitting
- more specialised drug abuse services
- anticoagulant monitoring
- more specialised alcohol abuse services.

It is anticipated that in the future changes will be made to the new GMS contract.

Personal Medical Services contract

Primary care organisations can use a locally agreed arrangement with practices, namely the Personal Medical Services (PMS) contract. This enables GPs to be offered salaried appointments, which is useful when it is difficult to recruit and retain them using the GMS contract.

PMS contract terms are decided between the PCT and the GP to tailor services to local need. Almost half of the GPs in the UK now work to PMS contracts.

Alternative Provider Medical Services (APMS)

Under the APMS arrangements, PCTs can contract with non-NHS organisations (voluntary or commercial sector providers) to supply primary medical services. They may also contract with secondary care organisations or other PCTs to provide these services.

Finance

Since April 2004 there have been many changes in general practice finances and funding. Many of the forms for items-of-service fees are no longer used. These include the following:

- claims for night visits
- minor surgery
- contraception
- temporary residents
- holiday vaccination
- emergency treatment

- new patient registration fees
- child health surveillance.

GP practices have been linked electronically to the PCO, and the items-of-service link is required in the new GMS contract to record services to unregistered patients (e.g. temporary residents), emergency treatment and immediately necessary treatments.

Since 2004, practices have been paid by a Global Sum which incorporates all of the above items of service in a yearly assessment that covers the expenses and profits related to the delivery of essential and additional services. The Global Sum payable to a practice is based on the number of patients registered with the practice, taking into account age range and the relative workload and costs that its patients represent as quantified by the Carr–Hill formula. Quarterly figures are submitted to the PCT for cervical screening and temporary residents. The Global Sum also includes the cost of staff salaries, for which general practitioners are now responsible.

Quality and Outcomes Framework

The level of quality achieved by GP practices is agreed with the PCO. Under the Quality and Outcomes Framework (QOF), practices agree their quality aspiration with the PCO. Aspiration payments are based on 60% of their previous year's level of achievement, and are paid over 12 equal monthly instalments. Audits are conducted to confirm other figures required by the Department of Health (e.g. data on diabetes, hypertension and asthma).

Forms in general practice

The only forms now completed in general practice are for patient registration (GMS1). Claims for vaccine are forwarded to the Prescription Pricing Authority. Receptionists may be asked for forms for exemption from prescription charge (FP92A) for medical conditions, or for maternity exemption forms (FW8).

When handling claim forms and target sheets, it is important to be systematic, and therefore it is preferable not to work on reception duties at the same time, trying to fit in the paperwork between other tasks. Paperwork requires a different set of skills to those used when receiving patients. If a receptionist works a busy morning shift on the reception desk it will be almost impossible to switch from pressured reception duties to calmly working through a pile of papers without a transitionary period – a cup of coffee, popping out to the shops for some fresh air, or a chat – to wind down from the pressure.

Box 9.1

RECEPTION DESK DUTIES	CLERICAL DUTIES
Require the ability to juggle many important priorities at once	Require a systematic orderly approach
Answering the telephone, controlling surgery flow and dealing with queries are 'demand-driven' activities	Processing massive piles of paper requires self-motivation – 'self-driven'

Note: It is appreciated that the duties of receptionists do vary considerably from one practice to another, and that they may not all be involved in completing and recording claim forms. In some medical practices this function is performed by the practice manager or administrator. Practices are linked electronically to their local PCT.

Practice income

Income to the practice is derived both from NHS sources and from private sources (e.g. medical attendant reports for insurance companies are a private source).

The new GMS contract specifies the circumstances in which GPs can charge patients a private fee. These are as follows:

- for a statutory body for the purpose of that body's statutory function

- for employers or schools for routine medical examinations

- for non-primary medical services in a nursing home

- for medico-legal examinations after road traffic accidents

- for attending a police station to examine a detainee

- for preparing a variety of medico-legal reports

- for travel immunisations that are not remunerated under the contract

- for prescribing drugs for foreign travel

- for medical examination for exemption from requirement to wear a seatbelt.

It is important that all sources of income are properly documented and claimed. The role of the receptionist in ensuring that services given are recorded and claimed for cannot be overestimated. The receptionist is the person who deals with the patients, is aware of what the doctor says he or she has done for a specific patient, and is therefore the pivotal person who ensures that claims are made or invoices are raised. The receptionist may not be required to do these tasks but to ensure that someone else has the necessary information to be able to do so.

However, there will be occasions when a receptionist is asked to advise a patient about what payment is required, to receive the payment and issue a receipt. Information about current fees should be kept readily to hand, together with printed receipts that only need to have the name of the patient, service given, date, amount paid and signature filled in by hand. The payment should then be passed to the appropriate person for banking.

Although most doctors are aware that private fees are a significant supplement to their income, some are reluctant to talk to patients about the fee for their services. Staff should also be aware that sums received from patients (large or small, cheque or cash) must all be passed through the practice accounts. Private fees are not a 'perk' – the Inland Revenue has been known to trace payments back over a number of years and claim back tax on them.

As in all of the other aspects of general medical practice, the receptionist has a vital role to play in the financial success of a practice by cutting down on unnecessary wastage and expense, and ensuring that all income is claimed and processed promptly.

GMS1: family doctor services registration

This is to be used:

- for an application to join a family doctor's list by a patient, child or someone who is unable to complete the form themselves

- for an application to join the NHS organ donor register.

At the practice

1 *Doctor to whom details of treatment given should be sent* – in the case of armed services personnel, this space should be used to record the current medical centre.

2 *Authorised signature* – ensure that the declaration is read before signing.

3 *Practice stamp* – this is a space for the practice stamp or for entering the name of the practice.

4 *Clinical records* – use the space provided to record details of treatment given, including if appropriate the type of vaccination/immunisation. These details will be passed on to the patient's home doctor.

5   *In case of queries* – enter the name of the doctor who should be contacted in case of queries by the patient's home doctor, and enter the practice address or stamp.

6   Do not write on this area, as it will affect the legibility of the patient's details on the reverse side of the form.

Receptionists may be asked for a self-certification form, which patients may complete when they have been off sick for four days or more.

Verification visits

The PCT in the past has undertaken post-payment verification of claims visits, but these have now stopped, although there may be an occasional visit to one or two surgeries in a PCT area each year.

PCT inspections

PCTs now inspect GP practices once a year, which may involve asking receptionists how they deal with difficult patients, or patients who collapse in the surgery. Receptionists may be asked what advice they would give over the phone in various circumstances, and when they would call an ambulance. PCT inspections can take from half a day to a full day, depending on the size of the practice. These inspections may be carried out less frequently in subsequent years.

Scotland

The new GMS contract in Scotland means that GPs working in Scotland will be rewarded to reflect the special needs and circumstances of the population. Devolution has resulted in the development of different health policies in Scotland to those in the rest of the UK.

Scottish Allocation Formula (SAF)

The SAF enables the distribution of resources to GP practices on the basis of the particular needs of the practice population. It is a population-based formula which reflects the following:

*   the age–sex structure of the practice population (demography)

- the additional needs of the practice population (morbidity and deprivation)

- the rurality and remoteness of the practice population.

The Scottish weighting formula provides an accurate indication of the socio-economic status of the Scottish population, using a deprivation and mortality index which is based on the following indicators:

- the unemployment rate

- the proportion of elderly people claiming income support

- the standardised mortality rate among people under the age of 65 years

- households with two or more areas of deprivation.

To identify any additional costs needed to provide GMS in remote and rural areas, a further weighting is applied based on the following indicators:

- the population density

- the population sparsity (the percentage of people living in settlements of less than 500 residents)

- the percentage of patients attracting road-mileage payments.

The SAF allocates a Global Sum based on Scottish factors and data.
   One of the advantages of the new GMS contract is that rural communities can enjoy the benefits as well as the urban practice population.

Inducement practitioners (IPs)

Under the new GMS contract, IPs have the following options:

- independent contractor status with a Global Sum, minimum practice income guarantee (MPIG), quality payments and enhanced services payments

- a salaried option

- the non-GMS contractual alternatives.

Out-of-hours services

In Scotland the aim is to ensure continuity of out-of-hours services by redesigning an integrated service which will enable nearly all GP practices to opt out of out-of-hours provision. However, a few isolated practices may have to continue to provide out-of-hours services for the time being, but it is anticipated that in the future they will be able to opt out altogether.

Wales

Generally speaking, the agreements contained within the new GMS contract apply to Welsh practices. The main areas of difference between the Welsh version of the contract and that for other countries in the UK are as follows:

- flexibility and funding arrangements with regard to premises development

- the agreement of Wales-wide arrangements for some of the direct and national enhanced services

- the information management and technology (IM&T) programme

- quality payments using Welsh disease prevalence data and Welsh average list sizes.

Premises flexibility

There is a Welsh GMS Premises Fund held by the National Assembly for Wales. Local Health Boards guarantee baseline funding to support agreed projects. GPs in collaboration with their Local Health Boards have to apply to the Assembly for the funding required in their Estate Strategies.

Development of health services

The new GMS contract outlines national arranagements to co-ordinate and facilitate the development of schemes to maximise the benefits of health service provision to patients and alternative models of service provision within general practice. The Assembly, led by the Primary Care Division, will undertake this.

Wales-wide arrangements for some of the direct and national enhanced services

The Welsh target with regard to access to GMS is that patients will be able to access an appropriate member of the primary care team within 24 hours of requesting an appointment, and much sooner than this in an emergency.

Direct and national enhanced services

Payment or central funding has been agreed for the following:

- direct enhanced services for influenza immunisation for patients under 65 years of age who are in the at-risk group
- quality information-directed enhanced services
- national enhanced services for anticoagulant monitoring and near-patient testing
- national enhanced services for patients who are drug abusers.

Quality payments

Disease prevalence is factored into clinical quality payments on a country-specific basis. GPs in Wales are paid according to Welsh prevalence data.

Northern Ireland

GPs in Northern Ireland have in the past had similar terms of service to the rest of the UK, although the Department of Health and Social Services has not been bound to accept the recommendations of the Doctors and Dentists Review Body, and the Northern Ireland General Practitioners Committee (GPC) is an autonomous committee.

The new GMS contract has marked a change in relationships, and the Northern Ireland GPC was represented in the UK negotiating team for the first time.

Northern Ireland has not suffered the recruitment and retention crisis that has been experienced elsewhere in the UK.

Essential and additional services

It appears that GP practices in Northern Ireland do not wish to avail themselves of the opportunity to opt out of additional services on the basis of workload pressure. Northern Ireland is readily able to recruit principals, and list sizes are smaller than in England and Wales.

Enhanced services

Northern Ireland has very long waiting-lists (longer than in the rest of the UK). One of the aims of the new GMS contract is to encourage the transfer of work from secondary care to primary care, thereby placing enhanced services in an ideal position to benefit from the contract.

GP practices agree an access target with their Board, and have another year or so to work towards the target of access to a primary care professional within 48 hours.

Quality and Outcomes Framework

Most practices in Northern Ireland are well placed to obtain a significant income from the quality framework. Quality points are weighted for prevalence – Northern Ireland has a higher prevalence in some disease areas (e.g. coronary heart disease).

Out-of-hours services

The new GMS contract gave GPs the opportunity to opt out of their out-of-hours duties from January 2005. Northern Ireland has a network of out-of-hours co-operatives and a commercial provider in Belfast. There are many more contacts in the out-of-hours period than in England, and they do not have support services such as NHS Direct, NHS 24 and walk-in centres. Most GPs have opted out. This has resulted in a decrease in the number of GPs providing out-of-hours services, and other primary care professionals (nurses, social workers and pharmacists) now deliver these services.

Flexible working

Unlike the rest of the UK, Northern Ireland does not have a problem with filling vacancies. It has around 1100 GPs and some vocationally trained GPs who work as locums, some of whom are seeking posts as principals. The GMS contract encourages flexibility in career options, which could lead to an increase in salaried GPs and part-time working, with some GPs working for out-of-hours providers.

10

Using information technology

What's in the box: basic terminology

<table>
<tr><td colspan="2">Box 10.1</td></tr>
<tr><td>Hardware</td><td>Physical components of the system, such as display screens, printers, keyboard, mouse, disks, etc.</td></tr>
<tr><td>Software</td><td>A set of programmed instructions in the computer which enable it to respond to input of information, and demands to change it, store it or print it out in various forms</td></tr>
<tr><td>CPU</td><td>The CPU, or central processor unit, is the part of the system that performs arithmetic operations and controls the storage, display, communication and manipulation of information. It is the part of the machine that is closest to a 'brain'</td></tr>
<tr><td>VDU</td><td>The screen that is used to display information held on the computer</td></tr>
<tr><td>Keyboard</td><td>A device like a typewriter for entering information into a computer. Many specialised systems use non-standard keyboards or make extensive use of special function keys to save typing effort</td></tr>
<tr><td>Mouse</td><td>A small hand-operated pointer which the user moves on a pad to move an arrow on the screen. Clicking a button on the mouse activates a number of operations without the need to type in text</td></tr>
</table>

Printer	A device that prints text and diagrams held on the computer on to paper. Older machines work like typewriters and are noisy and slow. Newer types work more like photocopiers or paint sprayers, and are much faster and quieter
Disk	Information cannot be permanently stored in the CPU. Usually it is stored on magnetic disk or tape. Tape is used for long-term secure storage and disks are used for information that is in constant use
Floppy disk	A disk which can be inserted into one computer to download and store data and which may be read by another computer. Most are 3.5 inches in diameter and contained in a rigid plastic case
Hard disk	A disk that is permanently held in the CPU and is used to store information needed on a permanent basis. Hard disks can hold many hundred times the information which can be stored by a floppy disk
Workstation	The work area where a computer operator works. Health and safety legislation gives details of how work-stations should be designed
Terminal	A machine that is capable of entering and retrieving information from a multi-user computer system. It may be a computer in its own right or, more usually, just a keyboard and screen
Network	When many people need to use the same computer system, several terminals can be linked together with cables. This, and the software needed for communication with a central CPU, is called a network
Byte	The measure of information that a computer can store. A byte is equivalent to a single text character, and one megabyte is equal to one million bytes. The more bytes of memory a computer or disk has, the more information it can store

How a computer works

It is not necessary to understand fully how computers work in order to operate the systems in use in GP practices, clinics and hospitals. The following brief outline is given merely for interest.

The central processor unit uses a system of on–off switches to hold information in a memory. Each number or character is expressed as a sequence of on or off states in a group of switches which together form a *byte*. As the operator enters information into the computer, it is translated into a machine-readable form and stored in the *random access memory* (RAM). This process is controlled by the computer's internal *operating system*. This is the raw material which is worked on by the computer's *application software*, which tells the machine how to display and manipulate the data to achieve the operator's needs, and how to interpret the instructions given by the operator.

The most common types of software are *word processors*, which enable the user to write documents, edit and print them. Most have facilities to store lists of names and addresses and insert these into one of a series of previously written standard letters. Routine correspondence can be produced far more efficiently in this way. Individual parts of a document can also be edited without the need for wholesale retyping. Importantly, information stored on one computer within a system (e.g. a patient administration system) can be imported on to another without the need to retype it.

Databases are applications designed to hold a lot of information about a series of people or things. An individual record (e.g. a patient) contains a variety of *fields* which may contain general text such as name, address and details of medical conditions. The field could have a specialised or limited range of values such as a postcode, date, or male or female, or it could be a code obtained from a published table such as diagnostic codings for different medical conditions. These codes are much easier for a computer system to analyse than is free text, which really needs a human brain to interpret it.

Spreadsheets are particularly suitable for arranging in order, displaying and performing calculations on mathematical data. They are commonly used to analyse treatments given to a large number of patients, or to calculate and report on budgets and expenditure. A typical small spreadsheet is shown in Table 10.1.

Table 10.1 Projected quarterly expenditure on staff training

Expenditure	First quarter	Second quarter	Third quarter	Fourth quarter
Staff time	£1287	£10 663	£7287	£5288
Expenses	£325	£8825	£8350	£3000
Total	£1612	£19 488	£15 637	£8288

Computers in general practice

General practice today is a highly complex organisation, and it is doubtful whether management of its administration can be effectively handled without information technology (IT).

Information technology in general practice has developed in a somewhat unsystematic way since the 1970s, and the General Practice Research Database (GPRD), previously known as VAMP, was one of the methods used to assess workloads for the new GMS contract.

The countries of the UK have differed in the information technology systems that they have used. In Scotland, the most widely used system (which is still in use today) is the GPASS, which was provided free of charge in Scotland and Northern Ireland until 1999. Elsewhere the cost of information technology in general practice was reimbursed under Government schemes.

GP systems developed based on GPs' contractual needs, but it was the electronic registration of patients and items-of service claims that led to health authorities establishing electronic links with practices. The Government has since standardised the systems, and the GMS contract gives the Government control both centrally and locally via PCOs to drive the information management and technology (IM&T) agenda.

With the advent of NHS intranets, the system has become linked with PCTs, providers of care and sources of clinical information. The new NHS number in England and Wales, and its equivalent in Northern Ireland and Scotland, is used to identify patients electronically for the following purposes:

- registration – including inclusion of new patients, and removal of patients from the list

- communication with the local PCT, secondary care and community sectors

- payment (for the Quality and Outcomes Framework)

- PCO financial planning

- needs assessment – for both central government and PCOs

- giving out-of-hours organisations access to practice medical records when treating patients

- Accident and Emergency access to GP records to assist in patient care and treatment

- electronic prescribing.

The integrated IM&T service means that the GP system is part of an NHS-wide system. Integration fits into the Government's Integrated Care

Records Service with appropriate benefits to patients in providing a better and more efficient health service.

Patient benefits through computerisation

A computerised appointments system overcomes the difficulties of manual appointment books (e.g. illegible handwriting, pages messy with cancellations, two people not being able to use the book at the same time, handwritten surgery lists for pulling out records, are all circumvented).

Reference was made to using IT for written communication in Chapter 3. Secretaries and receptionists are now able to use a word-processing package to generate mailmerged letters or letters to patients. Spreadsheets can be used either to collect data (for display in tables, graphs and pie charts) or to present doctor and staff rotas.

Desktop publishing software can be used to generate leaflets, posters and handouts.

Technology can save time for some tasks. For others it does not save time, but it does make it possible to produce professional-looking documents (e.g. practice leaflets, charts and posters).

For those who enjoy using a computer, it is essential that the computer does not become a barrier between the patient and the secretary or receptionist. Remember that it is as rude to continue to input or extract data as it is to continue to talk to a colleague or take a telephone call without acknowledging the presence of a patient.

The major disadvantage of IT in the practice is when the system 'goes down'. The increased efficiency then disappears and returning to manual systems, no matter how temporarily, results in unavoidable delays and disruption.

Age–sex register and patient information

These are basic patient data which are put on to the computer. Secretaries and receptionists will receive specific training in the use of their practice's information system.

The importance of inputting data accurately cannot be overstated, as this information will be of vital importance to the practice's activities. Remember, too, always to include the postcode. This is a vital piece of information and it should be cross-checked with the medical record in your possession.

You should be aware of the requirements of the Data Protection Act, and you must respect the security and confidentiality of patient information at all times.

Registration data

These data are of immense value. They include the following information about registration status:

- the date on which the patient was registered with the practice
- the date on which the patient was accepted onto the doctor's list
- the date on which the patient was included on a GP's patient list.

They will also indicate the category and date of a patient's removal from a doctor's list (e.g. when moving out of the area, or on death).

Repeat prescriptions

A computerised system can save much of the receptionist's time by obviating the need to retrieve patient files and other manually held prescribing information. In addition:

- it produces a legible, printed and accurate prescription
- it places a time limit on the issue of repeat prescriptions
- it monitors the rate and consumption of drugs
- it updates the repeat prescription record
- it easily identifies patients who are on a particular medication.

Screening and recall

The ability of a computer to search rapidly on the basis of specific criteria can allow a practice to identify certain groups of patients, including those selected for information (e.g. asthmatics, hypertensives, diabetics, etc.), who would benefit from additional care and those who are considered to be 'at risk'.

The computer can also help with the following:

- crisis intervention
- the control of chronic diseases
- preventive medicine.

Diagnoses and morbidity

A computer has the capacity and speed to extract and analyse data on any topics of particular interest to the practice (e.g. to analyse morbidity and treatment within the practice). The latest Royal College of General Practitioners (RCGP) coding system has been developed with a view to collecting these types of data from as many practices as possible.

Social recording

Computer systems are also capable of recording information on height/weight/smoking and alcohol-related habits in order to provide the PCOs with statistics. This information is automatically included in the patients' records.

Electronic links and other developments

Electronic links convey correspondence, such as patient test results and consultant letters, directly between the sender's and the recipient's computer systems. The electronic linkage is made by using public and private telephone networks. The technical term used for the transfer of such data is electronic data interchange (EDI), where the sender's information is converted into a form which can be conveyed through telephone lines via a modem.

The advantages of electronic links are as follows:

- less duplication of tasks (e.g. patient registration)
- fewer transcription errors (where data are entered only once)
- reduced paperwork (form-filling)
- easier and faster access to information.

The main applications of electronic links are as follows:

- links with the PCT for the exchange of patient registration information
- links with local hospitals for the exchange of:
  - patient referral correspondence between GPs and consultants
  - laboratory test results and reports and requests from GPs.

Electronic medicine

Technology is advancing so rapidly in the health service that it is difficult to keep up to date with exactly what is going on. You will have found that in the workplace your computers are being used increasingly for recording of data, and that they are linked to your NHS trust. The terms 'NHSnet' and 'telemedicine' are now commonplace.

Box 10.2   More computer 'jargon'

Internet	A framework which allows the exchange of information between computers
Internet provider	A company which provides access to the Internet. There are a number of providers and a choice of ways to pay for the connection
Website	A source of information on the Internet on many topics and subjects, arranged on individual pages
Network interface	The part of the computer that enables information to be transmitted over a telephone line
Modem	Hardware that allows the computer to 'talk' over a telephone line. It may be used as a network interface

---

What e-health will do

With the reality of e-health dawning, patients and healthcare professionals should all see an improved and more responsive service that brings about fast and easy access to vital information.

NHS Direct online

NHS Direct online is the gateway to health advice and information on the Internet. It includes an easy-to-use guide to treating common symptoms at home, and links to thousands of sources of help and advice.

National Electronic Library for Health (NeLH)

NeLH is a NHS website for health professionals, providing up-to-date best practice information on diagnosis and treatment.

Telemedicine Information Service

The Telemedicine Information Service provides a directory giving details of and contacts for around 120 UK telemedicine projects. This service is provided by the British Library in conjunction with a healthcare computing group. Individuals who do not have access to the Internet can interrogate the database by telephone.

Telemedicine

Telemedicine is the term given to electronic means of delivering health services. It allows doctors many miles apart to communicate both with one another and with patients, and to conduct live consultations from all over the world via the Internet. By adding a camera to the system, video conferencing or video telemedicine becomes possible, whereby all parties involved can view each other, thus simulating a 'live' consultation.

There are certain areas where telemedicine could be particularly useful, such as the treatment of terminally ill patients at home. Videophones would enable patients, carers or relatives to communicate with clinicians without having to make the journey to hospital. Telemedicine could also be useful for supporting medical staff in crisis situations, enabling them to obtain expert advice from remote links.

Future implementation plans

The NHS information strategy stipulates that all trusts should have electronic prescribing systems in place by 2005, which will help to prevent the types of errors that may occur with handwritten prescriptions in hospitals.

New technology will enable cross-matching of blood samples to be performed electronically, thereby saving staff time and money, as well as facilitating the provision of blood for trauma victims. Hospital laboratories are being given the go-ahead to move towards electronic cross-matching (EXR).

Computers in hospitals

Computerisation of records in hospitals works well because there is a great deal of information to be stored and consulted, information is required by a variety of people at different times and in different locations, much of the information needs to be sorted or changed, and complex analysis of data is required.

This is not because computers are 'clever'. They are not – they have no real intelligence or ability to think of solutions. However, computers can process vast amounts of data at incredible speed with virtually no errors. A 'computer error' is almost always due to a human operator doing the wrong thing or the computer's programmer setting it up wrongly in the first place.

The main systems used in hospitals are the patient administration system (PAS), word-processing, and record storage in pathology, X-ray and pharmacy departments. Other major systems are used in finance and personnel departments, estates management and supplies, and are being introduced into nursing and theatre management.

Patient administration systems (PAS)

The potential of computers has long been exploited in hospitals in the area of patient administration. There are many versions used by different hospitals, but all of them have the same component parts (*see* Box 10.3).

Box 10.3

Patient index	Records of the personal details of every patient
Admissions, discharges and transfers	A record of each patient's history of time spent in the hospital as an inpatient or outpatient, with particular consultants or in a particular department
Waiting-lists	Names and dates of referral of all patients waiting for inpatient and/or outpatient treatment
Outpatients	A system to manage appointments and correspondence associated with outpatient clinics
GP index	A list of the names and addresses of all of the local GPs

---

Nursing management systems

Increasingly, hospitals are being equipped with computer systems to help nurses to plan and keep track of the nursing care of patients. Patients' details are retrieved from PAS, and a detailed plan of their expected care is prepared. Care given is recorded on the system to help to co-ordinate the work of the team. Patient dependency levels can be predicted from the care plans, and nurse rosters are drawn up to match needs.

Order communication systems

In most hospitals, ordering portering services, pathology tests, supplies of materials or repairs to buildings or equipment must be done by telephone or by completing a form, often with multiple copies and requiring posting to the relevant department. This can take a long time and involve much duplication of effort. An order communications (or 'order-comms') system allows ordering departments to send requests for services directly to the department, and to receive confirmation of orders or the results of tests directly.

Hospital information support system (HISS)

The trend among hospitals with well-established computer systems is to integrate them into one powerful scheme called a hospital information support system (HISS). Such a system allows every department's computer system to communicate with those of other departments, to transfer information and to generate reports.

Information, management and technology

The NHS is investing vast sums of money in information technology over the next three years in a programme to completely revise and update its current IT systems with integrated patient health information and records.

It is intended that these new systems will:

• change the way in which care is delivered

• allow the effective use of resources

• result in improved quality of care.

The Wanless Report (*see* Appendix 14) has recommended the following for information technology in the NHS:

- improved management of IT implementation, including a national programme
- doubling the IT budget and ensuring that funding is not used to subsidise other services
- stringent, centrally managed national standards for IT.

What is happening now?

National Programme for Information Technology

In April 2005 the National Programme for Information Technology (NPIT) was amalgamated as an agency of the Department of Health, and it is now called *NHS Connecting for Health*. This new agency is based in Leeds.

NHS Connecting for Health anticipates that, over the next ten years, it will connect England's general practitioners to its hospitals, and it will enable patients to access their health and care information. Information will be swiftly transferred and will include the following:

- healthcare records
- prescription information
- appointment details
- up-to-date research (accessible to both professionals and patients).

This information will support patient choice and will allow hospital outpatient appointments to be made at a time and place convenient to the individual patient.

Significant differences and improvements in the service can be classified into four key areas as follows:

- underpinning IT infrastructure with sufficient connectivity and broadband capacity
- electronic transmission of prescriptions
- electronic appointment systems and booking
- electronic care records service.

Commercial suppliers are working together to develop and integrate IT systems to be used on a national basis, such as the NHS Care Records Service.

Electronic booking (Choose and Book)

The Choose and Book system will underpin the Government's policy of giving patients greater choice, enabling them to choose which hospital to attend at a date and time convenient to them. New software will enable GPs and other primary care staff to book hospital or clinic appointments while the patient is still at the surgery.

As a result, clinicians will be able to readily track referrals and, where appropriate, discuss cases by email. This will give consistent and accurate referral data without the need to wait for paper correspondence. It is expected that Choose and Book will both reduce the number of non-attenders at hospital clinics and improve clinical governance.

The implementation of Choose and Book should have occurred by December 2005, but provision has been slower than anticipated. As a result, the Government has offered PCTs a financial incentive to encourage GP practices to install the system as soon as possible.

NHS Care Records Service

The NHS Care Records Service is a single electronic record system to which all care providers have access. This is of vital importance as patients attend various institutions at different times, consulting and meeting different healthcare professionals, including GPs and primary care staff, secondary care clinicians and other professionals, social services and the independent sector.

The NHS Care Records Service will connect NHS trusts and GPs in a single national system, and will provide all patients in England with an individual, secure electronic record that gives details of all key treatments in both the health service and social care. All doctors, nurses and related healthcare professionals who have a legitimate need to access patient information will be able to do so 24 hours a day, seven days a week. This service will be used for the following:

- routine single and multiple episodes of care

- emergency and unscheduled care

- care pathways (e.g. National Service Frameworks)

- telecare and services such as NHS Direct.

The first phase was completed in 2005, will include booking outpatient appointments and enabling health and social care professionals to view basic patient information.

The aim is that the second phase will be completed in 2006 and will enable healthcare professionals to access more detailed patient records and make electronic requests for X-rays, pathology and diagnostic imaging. It will also give information on emergency and out-of-hours treatments.

Two further phases will complete the project by 2010, and will give full integration of the health and social care systems.

Electronic transmission of prescriptions (ETP)

ETP enables prescriptions to be transferred electronically to pharmacists nominated by the patient, and to be sent automatically to the Prescription Pricing Authority. ETP will improve patient safety by reducing errors, will provide a better service at the point of prescribing and dispensing, and will reduce adverse drug reactions. It ensures that full prescription information becomes part of each patient's NHS record and becomes progressively available during 2005.

The New National Network (N3)

N3 is replacing the communications network, NHSnet. It will link all NHS locations electronically for the first time. N3 has sufficient connectivity and broadband capacity to meet the NHS's current and anticipated future needs. It will enable clinicians to send high-quality images to specialists for remote diagnostics, and it will allow secure clinical messaging. N3 will therefore facilitate video conferencing and remote working.

Connections to N3 have already started, and will take about three years to complete.

Health and Social Care Information Service

The Health and Social Care Information Service is a new special health authority which was set up in 2005. It aims to facilitate information flow across the whole system and to improve the credibility of reported information, while reducing the burden of information collection. It has taken over some of the information-related functions of the former NHS Information Authority, as well as the statistics and information management function of the Department of Health.

More of the electronic NHS: what's new?

Contact

Contact is a national email directory service for NHS staff which has been specially developed to meet the British Medical Association's requirements for clinical email between NHS organisations. It provides a national directory of individuals working in the NHS, and includes the following information:

- email addresses
- telephone numbers

- name and address of the individual's NHS organisation/department
- job roles
- specialties.

Staff are given an email address that will move with them if they change their job and/or location in the NHS.

NHSweb

Websites can be hosted exclusively on the NHSnet for NHS use, and are then described as being on NHSweb as opposed to being on the World Wide Web. NHSweb also hosts the intranet to individual NHS organisations. Users who are connected to other networks are 'blocked' and cannot access sites on NHSweb.

nhs.uk

nhs.uk is the official gateway to NHS organisations on the Internet. It provides both NHS staff and the public with information at a local and national level, including directories of all NHS organisations and the services that they offer.

NHS number

The new NHS number is a unique identifier that provides the link between a patient's records (both electronic and manual) across the NHS. It is a vital part of the move to achieve the electronic health record, and it enables information to be collated in order to build a complete and comprehensive record of a person's health. Everyone is now given an NHS number from birth.

NHS Strategic Tracing Service (NSTS)

This is a national database of people, places and organisations. Its main function is to trace NHS numbers and confirm the personal details of the patients identified by these numbers, including the following:

- date of birth
- sex
- death (where applicable)
- GP and practice address.

This information is provided by PCTs and the Registrar of Births and Deaths.

The NSTS is scheduled to be taken over from June 2006, when demographic information management will be handled by the NHS Care Records Service.

NHS Careers

This is a 24-hour helpline website that provides information on careers in the NHS in England. It also provides literature and supporting services for NHS employees, as well as for schools, colleges and careers advisers.

NHS Jobs

NHS Jobs is a new NHS website that provides information about jobs, and it is linked with the NHS careers site. There are over 400 NHS organisations across England registered on the service.

Primary Care Information Service (PRIMIS)

PRIMIS offers free help and support to primary care organisations to enable them to make maximum use of the clinical computer systems. It works through locally funded facilitators, and provides GP practices with training in information management skills and recording for data quality, as well as analysis of data quality. It also provides a comparative analysis service that is focused on key clinical topics, feedback and interpretation of results and support in developing action plans to improve data quality. NPIT is currently procuring a new service that will build on the success of PRIMIS after the current contract with Nottingham University has expired.

Box 10.4 Some useful acronyms

CHDGP	Collecting Health Data from General Practice
CTI	Computers in Teaching Initiative
EHR	Electronic Health Record
IM&T	Information, Management and Technology
LIS	Local Implementation Strategy
NeLH	National Electronic Library for Health
RHI	Regional Head of Information
RFA	Requirements for Accreditation of GP Systems

Getting the best from the computer

The importance of inputting data accurately cannot be overstated, as this information is to be used by healthcare professionals when treating and caring for patients, and for statistical analysis and planning, budgeting, contract monitoring and invoicing for services. Information held on the computer must be regularly cross-checked with that held on medical records, and it should be amended as necessary. Incorrect information about a patient can lead to important letters or test results going astray.

Problems which arise in hospitals are frequently caused by out-of-date addresses, either because the patient has moved house or changed GP, or both. Other problems arise from incomplete details, or temporary addresses entered as permanent ones (e.g. when a person is taken ill when visiting relatives). Errors in this information can be very costly to the hospital, since if the bill is sent to the wrong health authority or GP fundholder, they are unlikely to pay.

The barrier created by the computer

Computer systems usually require the input of patient information in a specific sequence, which may not be the same as that which the patient wants to give. Sometimes the computer is slow to respond if many people are using it. Receptionist staff frequently have to deal with a patient on the telephone, another in person, and call up details on to their screen, all at the same time. Both the patient and the receptionist may start to feel that they are the servant of the computer, rather than the other way round.

To overcome these difficulties it is important to explain to the patient what is happening (especially when you are on the telephone), and to develop a sequence of questions which gives the information you need in the correct order. This often requires a good deal of practice and discussion with colleagues before it works really well.

Maintaining security

There are four main risks to be guarded against when using computer systems:

• unauthorised access to information held on computer

• loss of information due to mechanical failure

- theft of machinery
- spoiling of information by computer viruses.

Preventing unauthorised access

Information about people that is held on computer is governed by the Data Protection Act. It should only be used for the purpose for which it was collected and should not be revealed to unauthorised individuals. Where password systems exist, these must be used, and passwords should never be shared or revealed to others. Computer screens should face away from public areas. Terminals should not be left unattended showing data or even 'logged on' to a system, since anyone may then gain access.

Backing up – keeping spare copies of information

If information has been stored on a computer's hard disk and it is lost due to mechanical failure or theft, a great deal of work will be needed to replace it. It is therefore extremely important to keep copies on a separate storage device. Taking such copies is known as *backing up,* and should be done daily. Staff using a multi-user system may find that this is done centrally by a system manager. Each night the latest data are copied on to large tape recorders.

Personal computers should be backed up either to a central back-up store via a hospital network, or to removable floppy disks or specially designed tape records (called tape streamers). Locally made back-up copies should be stored away from the computer in case of theft or fire.

Guarding against theft

Backing up is also important in case a computer is stolen. Such thefts from hospitals and healthcare premises are becoming increasingly common. All premises should be secure and kept locked. Machinery should be indelibly marked and preferably fastened to the desktop and alarmed with one of a variety of proprietary products. Computers should be housed away from public view wherever possible (e.g. away from windows without blinds).

Computer viruses

These are small programs designed to damage data held on computer. They are transferred from one machine to another when other files are copied, perhaps from floppy disk or by electronic connection. To guard against this, material should never be copied from a disk which has not been checked for viruses, nor should games and other such programs be copied on to work machines. Computer equipment and disks should be routinely checked for the presence of virus programs.

Illegal use of software

Commercial computer programs are protected by copyright. In general, a program can only be used on one computer unless a site licence has been purchased. The penalties for using programs which are not licensed are extremely high.

Computers and the law

Where medical records are stored on computer it is a requirement that computer-held material is at least as confidential as a paper record. Special care must be taken with computerised information, since it is possible to write programs which allow different people different levels of access. For example, it is possible to give a doctor access via the computer to all of the information that is held, whereas the clerk may only see certain material. Some staff will be allowed to change information, while others will have 'read only' access.

Data protection (*see* Chapter 4)

Organisations which record information on computer relating to identifiable living individuals must ensure that they comply with the provisions of the Data Protection Act. This Act applies to England, Wales, Scotland and Northern Ireland.

The Data Protection Act is based on eight principles, and is designed to ensure that information relating to an individual is obtained fairly, is kept up to date and is stored securely. The individual whose data are stored has rights of access enabling him or her to check the accuracy of the information. The Data Protection Registrar and the courts are empowered to require correction of inaccurate material if it is not undertaken voluntarily by the data user.

Useful websites and references

www.connectingforhealth.nhs.uk
www.library.nhs.uk/management
www.nelh.nhs.uk
NHS Confederation (2004) *Briefing 96. Electronic Booking – an initial guide to implementation*. NHS Confederation, London.
NHS Confederation (2004) *Briefing 1105. The NHS Care Records Service*. NHS Confederation, London.
www.nhs.uk
Department of Health (1998) *General Principles in the Use of the NHS Number*. Department of Health, London.
www.nhscareers.co.uk
www.jobsnhs.uk
www.primisnhs.uk

11

Medical terminology and clinical aspects

Introduction

Medical secretaries and receptionists, with their unique skills in dealing with doctors, other professionals and patients with tact and courtesy, will find that a knowledge of medical terminology will help them to carry out their duties in a more effective and efficient manner. Very often the words and phrases used by medical professionals are long, difficult and apparently obscure.

Medical terminology is based upon root words derived from Greek and Latin. To these roots may be added syllables that modify the meaning of the root word. An addition made to the front of a root is known as a *prefix*, and an addition at the end is known as a *suffix*. Over the years this principle has been modified in such a way that it can be applied to modern medical techniques. For example, the word 'gaster' (Greek) means 'stomach'. The root word used in medical terminology is 'gastr-o' and by adding the suffix 'itis', the word is modified to *gastritis*, meaning 'inflammation of the stomach'. By adding the suffix 'oscopy', we obtain the word *gastroscopy*, which means in this modified form 'visual inspection of the stomach' (by means of a gastroscope).

It is not intended to go into a detailed explanation of medical terminology here, but rather to point out that a limited knowledge of some root words, prefixes and suffixes will give a wider understanding of the medical vocabulary. Appendix 4 lists some of the most commonly used root words, prefixes and suffixes.

Medical abbreviations are also frequently used by professionals in healthcare, and again a knowledge of these will be of value (*see* Appendix 4).

Pathology and X-ray examinations

Medical secretaries and receptionists will find that doctors refer patients for pathological and other investigations and tests. An awareness of the most commonly used tests will not only contribute to the effectiveness of their day-to-day work, but will also make their job more interesting and fulfilling (*see* Appendix 4).

Prescribing and drugs

The supply, distribution and storage of drugs are controlled by a series of Acts of Parliament which are designed to control their sale and reduce their danger to life from sale by unqualified individuals.

Secretaries and receptionists will find that a knowledge of the drugs most frequently used by the medical practice or hospital consultant will be of value in their day-to-day work.

Receptionists in general practice have greater direct involvement with repeat prescribing for their patients, and will often have to deal with queries. However, the receptionist must have clear instructions and never be placed in the position of having to make medical decisions.

Components of a prescription

The following information must be included on every prescription issued by the prescriber, whether it is an NHS or private prescription. Without this information it is not possible for the pharmacist to dispense the drugs. Sometimes the writing on the prescription may be illegible, but this is not so common now that most prescriptions in general practice are computer generated.

Drug name

This may be written as the generic or approved name of the drug, or its trade or proprietary name. For example:

- salbutamol (generic)
- Ventolin (proprietary).

A number of commonly used drugs have been renamed in order to bring nomenclature in the UK into line with that in other countries. For example:

- bendrofluazide has been renamed bendroflumethiazide
- dothiepin has been renamed dosulepin.

See Appendix X in the current *British National Formulary*.

Form of prescribed drug

This refers to whether capsules, tablets, syrup, injection, ointment, etc. are required.

Strength

Many drugs are available in more than one strength, which must be specified.

Directions

Directions to the patient regarding the dosage of the medicine should be included. The *British National Formulary* recommends that directions should preferably be written in English, without abbreviation. However, some doctors still use Latin abbreviations (*see* Appendix 4; *see also* inside back cover of the *British National Formulary*).

Amount or quantity

A box on NHS prescription forms can be completed to indicate the number of days for which the treatment is to continue. If this is not used, the quantity to be dispensed should be included.

Problems with prescriptions

Medical receptionists and secretaries should be aware that problems can be caused by the following:

- missing information (e.g. strength of drug, missing form or type of drug, missing dose)
- incorrect or inaccurate information (e.g. incorrect name of drug) (similar drug names can cause problems – for instance, *chlorpropamide* which is used for treating diabetes and *chlorpromazine*, an antipsychotic drug)
- incorrect strength or incorrect dose
- amounts of medicine prescribed (patients often complain that they have run out of one medicine and still have some others left.

Remember that medicines come in different pack sizes – some in 28s, some in 30s, etc.).

Controlled drugs

The relevant legislation concerning controlled drugs is the Misuse of Drugs Regulations 1985 and subsequent amendments.

For controlled drugs there are rules for the following:

- who can possess and supply
- record keeping
- storage
- prescription writing.

Records

Secretaries and receptionists should understand that it is the doctor's duty to maintain a register, in an approved form, of the quantity of all controlled drugs obtained and supplied, including any administered personally, with names and addresses.

Storage

All controlled drugs in the custody of a doctor must be kept in a locked cupboard that can only be opened by the doctor or with his or her authority.

It is the doctor's responsibility to ensure that the controlled drugs cupboard is locked and the keys put safely away. The medical secretary or receptionist should make sure that this has been done.

Prescribing controlled drugs

Special rules apply to the prescribing of controlled drugs. A prescription for a controlled drug must:

- be written in ink, or otherwise so as to be indelible, and it must be signed and dated by the person issuing it with his or her usual signature
- be written by the person issuing it in his or her own handwriting
- specify the name and address of the person for whom it is intended
- specify the strength of the preparation, the dose to be taken and the quantity of the preparation in both words and figures.

An exception to these rules is phenobarbitone. Receptionists can write prescriptions for this, but the quantity must be written in both words and figures.

Some general medical practitioners in England and Wales use a special prescription form (FP10 (MDA)) for treatment of substance misusers by instalment with the controlled drugs *methadone* and *buprenopine* (Subutex). A total of 14 days' treatment by instalments may be prescribed.

Only medical practitioners who hold a special licence from the Home Secretary can prescribe the controlled drugs *cocaine*, *diamorphine* and *dipipanone* for addiction, although all general medical practitioners can still prescribe these drugs for relief of pain due to illness or injury, without a special licence.

At the time of going to press, the fourth report of the Shipman Inquiry (published in 2004) contained a number of recommendations on the regulation of controlled drugs in the community. The recommendations include tighter controls on the prescribing, dispensing, storage, inspection and disposal of controlled drugs. New limitations on prescribing rights and the introduction of special controlled-drug prescription forms have been proposed.

Repeat prescribing

The doctor is responsible for issuing the initial prescription to the patient, and for explaining what the preparation is and what it is intended to do, etc. The patient does not always remember this information, and will often discuss any problems with the receptionist or secretary.

Some patients are on regular drug regimes and are able to request repeat prescriptions without seeing the doctor before they run out of their medication. Repeat prescriptions are routinely generated with matching 'repeat-request' computer printouts.

In general practice, receptionists play a vital role in the repeat prescription procedure of the practice.

- They receive the requests from patients for a repeat of their medication.

- They will generate a repeat prescription on the practice computer to be signed by the doctor.

- A record is kept on the computer or in the patient's medical record (or both) of repeat prescribing.

- They will explain to the patient how to make the best use of the repeat prescription service offered by the practice (e.g. the procedures and system used – the use of cards, computer printouts, or telephone, fax or practice website requests for repeat prescriptions).

The repeat prescription system used by the medical practice is designed not only to make better use of the doctor's time, but also to suit the patient's needs. Every practice has its own system to ensure that patients obtain their prescriptions on a regular basis. Review dates are automatically included on 'repeat-request' printouts.

Many pharmacies now offer a repeat medication service which is operated in co-operation with local medical practices. Patients or carers who wish to take advantage of such a service must initiate requests for their repeat prescriptions to be directed to a particular pharmacy for dispensing. Reception staff are often responsible for placing these repeat prescriptions in bags provided by local pharmacies, which are collected on a regular basis by pharmacy employees. The ready-dispensed prescriptions are then collected by patients from the respective pharmacy, or are delivered to the housebound by arrangement. The role of the receptionist is very important for the smooth running of 'collection and delivery' repeat medication services.

Computer-generated prescriptions

All practices are now computerised and have a computer that generates repeat prescriptions. Although computer-generated prescriptions are accurate and time saving, secretaries and receptionists should realise that computers are only efficient if the correct information has been entered in the first place. Therefore, when entering details of patients' medication into the computer, always check that all of the information is there (e.g. that the right drug, its strength, the correct dose and quantity have been entered).

The same attention to detail is necessary when making amendments to existing drug records – for example, when doses have been changed following a clinical review of the patient and their medication by the medical practitioner. It is therefore extremely important that computer records are kept up to date with accurate data.

Sources of information

Doctors receive a great deal of information which is designed to help them when prescribing for their patients. Medical secretaries and receptionists will no doubt have access to the following useful sources of information:

- the *British National Formulary* (*BNF*)

- the *Monthly Index of Medical Specialities* (*MIMS*).

The *BNF*, which is published twice yearly, is an official and reliable source of accurate information on prescribing. It contains helpful guidance on prescription writing, emergency supplies of medicines and drug dependence. *MIMS* is sent to doctors each month. It is a good, 'user-friendly' information source, but printing errors may occasionally occur. Both publications provide details of constituents, manufacturers, packaging, net costs, etc., of every medicine that can be prescribed.

Branded or generic

Every drug that a doctor prescribes will fall into one of two categories:

- branded
- generic.

The term 'branded' refers to the proprietary name of a drug that is given by a manufacturer, whilst the term 'generic' means that the name is a general one which describes the pharmacological product. Both the *BNF* and *MIMS* give cross-referenced information on generic and brand-named products.

There is an increasing trend for medical practitioners to prescribe generic drugs, as they are often cheaper than their 'branded' or proprietary equivalents. Sometimes, as a result of practice policy, patients on repeat medication are 'switched' to generic drugs and need reassurance that their new medication has essentially the same action as the original 'branded' medication.

Practice prescribing policies

Prescribing analyses and costs (PACT)

Secretaries and receptionists in general practice will be aware that their practice prescribing policy to a certain extent reflects national and local guidelines.

The Prescription Pricing Authority (PPA) sends a statement each quarter giving information on what individual doctors and the whole practice are prescribing, how much is being spent on drugs, and how they compare locally and nationally with other doctors and practices. GP practices are given an indicative target cost to aim for, which is designed to encourage effective prescribing procedures. The local primary care trust, through its prescribing subcommittee or the equivalent, generates guidance for practices on prescribing, which also reflects the needs of the local population.

Practice formularies

There are many medicines and preparations available on prescription, a number of which are the same generic drug with a different proprietary name. Practices are reducing the number of drugs they prescribe and, where appropriate yet in the patient's best interests, will try to achieve the national approach.

The community pharmacist

Pharmacists, in common with general practitioners, have a contract with the NHS which clearly states their terms of service. This contract, together with the requirements of the Medicines Act, provides the framework within which pharmacists work.

The pharmacist is a professional person who will from time to time telephone a medical practice to speak to a doctor or a member of the team. This may be to query a prescription item or the frequency of its repeat. The receptionist or secretary should always immediately connect the pharmacist to the doctor, being aware that they are acting in accordance with legal and professional responsibility.

Most primary care trusts employ community pharmacists who are based in medical practices. Their role involves supporting the practice in achieving rational and cost-effective prescribing, for example by:

- advising on repeat-prescribing policies

- reviewing medication changes on patients' discharge from hospital

- assisting with the development of practice formularies.

All community pharmacists keep computerised records of medicines dispensed to patients, and are thus readily aware of potential problems.

Nurse prescribing

District nurses and health visitors are able to prescribe certain medicinal preparations, and a list of these may be found in the Nurse Prescribers' Formulary included in the *British National Formulary* (BNF), p. 834.

Independent nurse prescribers are nurses who have completed the necessary training and are authorised to prescribe from the Extended Formulary, also included in the BNF, p. 840. They can prescribe all 'General Sales List' and Pharmacy medicines (as prescribed by general practitioners), together with specified 'Prescription-Only Medicines'. In addition, they may prescribe all items included in the nurse prescribing list.

New developments in pharmacy

A new community pharmacy contract for England and Wales was implemented in April 2005. It consists of a national contract covering 'essential services' to be provided by all pharmacists, as well as optional 'advanced services'. The eight essential services are as follows:

- dispensing (eventually to include electronic transmission of prescriptions)
- repeat dispensing
- disposal of unwanted medicines
- promotion of healthy lifestyles
- signposting
- support for self-care
- support for people with disabilities
- clinical governance.

Once pharmacies have met the essential service requirements, they will be able to move on to providing advanced services such as the 'medicines use review' and 'prescription intervention service'.

Repeat dispensing schemes have been initiated to allow patients to obtain prescriptions from their GPs, which can then be dispensed by their pharmacists in several instalments. When patients, many with chronic conditions, collect their instalments, pharmacists have an opportunity to confirm that the prescription still meets their needs. These schemes have proved convenient for patients and waste of medicines has been reduced.

The *electronic transmission of prescriptions* has undergone extensive trials and NHS-wide standards have been developed to allow routine electronic transfer of prescriptions in the community as well as hospitals. Patients should benefit from easier ordering of repeat prescriptions while pharmacists will benefit from the new opportunities to use information technology to support their practice.

E-pharmacy developments allow people to consult their pharmacist electronically to seek advice, purchase over-the-counter medicines, and to make arrangements for the delivery of their dispensed prescriptions. The introduction of electronic prescribing will mean that a prescription can be transferred to a pharmacy electronically, thereby widening the dispensing choice available to patients.

Finally, prescribing rights have been extended to pharmacists, building on the success of nurse prescribing. Following the introduction of new legislation, a number of pharmacists have qualified as 'supplementary prescribers'. Prescribing pharmacists share responsibility for the continuing care of patients who have been clinically assessed by an independent prescriber.

Pharmacist prescribing might include pharmacists' involvement in anticoagulant clinics, where treatment requires careful monitoring and adjustment of doses. Adding a prescribing role to their existing responsibilities will enable pharmacists to provide a better and more efficient service to patients, especially those with long-term or chronic conditions.

12

Primary healthcare services and social services

Introduction

The Community Care Act provides a practical structure for managing patients in their own homes.

The Community Care Act gives patients or clients and/or their relatives an active part in deciding what care they receive, compared with the previous situation where the health authority and social services provided a range of services and the patient received the service deemed to be most appropriate for them by doctors, nurses, social workers or care managers.

Social care services look after the health and welfare of the population. Everyone is likely to become a client of social care services at one time or aonther, but some of the main groups include the following:

- children or families who are under stress
- people with disabilities
- people with emotional or psychological difficulties
- people with financial or housing problems
- others who need help with daily living activities.

Social care services deal with many issues and so can operate in many different settings. These services may be offered in hospitals or health centres, educational settings, community groups, residential homes, intermediate care institutions or people's own homes.

Care in the community includes both community nursing services and social services. As each patient is referred to the community nursing services (from a hospital, a general practitioner), an assessment is conducted with the patient, and with their relatives if they wish, in the home. A nursing care plan is agreed which is tailored to meet the needs of the patient. Typical services provided by community nurses would include giving injections (e.g. insulin to housebound diabetics), palliative care to patients who are dying, and dressings and removal of stitches after surgery, or blood samples or swabs for pathology. Patients do not make any personal contribution to the cost of their care (i.e. the service is free).

With social care, a care plan is agreed between the patient and the social worker. However, the patient's financial situation is also taken into account in order to work out the patient's contribution towards the cost. (Patients have made a contribution towards social services received for some time, and no one goes without a service they need simply because they cannot afford it.) Social services provide for children and families, the elderly, and patients with mental illness, learning difficulties, permanent disabilities and alcohol problems. To supplement care given by families, friends and neighbours, help may come from the following sources:

- social workers, home carers and meals on wheels
- sheltered housing, day centres, residential homes and nursing homes
- wardens and housing officers
- voluntary groups, visitors and churches.

These services play an important role in enabling people to be cared for at home.

Apart from meals on wheels, which delivers a hot cooked meal to the patient's home, luncheon clubs encourage patients to socialise, carer support groups encourage family members and friends to share their experiences and support one another, and information services help patients and families to know what is available to them. Simple practical help, such as assistance with bathing, light housework or preparing a meal, is now provided by home carers who are specially trained to do this work.

Further information about community nursing or social services provided in any particular area of the country will be available from local council offices who publish leaflets or via their website, outlining what they provide, to whom, and how to access the services.

The limit on funds for health and social care results in decisions being made about what service or care is received dependent on funds available. This concept is very difficult for a nation that has come to depend on a free health service which is available to all at the point of need. The reality of the situation is that the Government does not have a bottomless purse, so the responsibility for deciding who receives what care is being transferred to those who deal with the patients – doctors, healthcare and social care workers. Therefore the role of health professionals is changing from 'helping people' and responding to need, to include assessment and management, and offsetting need against available funds.

Dentists, opticians and pharmacists are also contracted to primary care trusts to provide their services.

Social care services are normally run by local councils, sometimes in conjunction with local NHS providers and organisations. Many councils often work together to run social care services.

Trusts and fundholding

The White Paper *Working for Patients* led to the reforms stated in the NHS and Community Care Act 1990, such as the 'internal market', where 'providers' of healthcare (hospitals, community services and ambulances) were separated from 'purchasers' (GPs and local health authorities). Purchasers were given a budget to enable them to purchase services from the providers.

This led to the emergence of NHS trusts, which enabled providers to be independent, self-managed, competitive providers of healthcare.

By 1995, trust status had been given to ambulance services. Their whole range of services, from transporting patients to hospital outpatient clinics, to emergency admissions, doctors' answering service, paging, community alarms and nursing answering service, are now managed against budgets with built-in standards of achievement (e.g. for patients being transported to a particular clinic, they will be picked up and returned within a specific time of their appointment so that they are not kept waiting at the hospital for hours on end).

Primary care trusts (*see also* Chapter 1)

Primary care trusts (PCTs) run primary and community services and commission care from a wide range of NHS and other providers. The Government has stated that it wishes the health service to be primary care led – that is, for primary care staff to have an overview of both hospital and community services as well as public health and well-being services and local authority provision.

The main functions of PCTs are to improve the health of the community, to develop primary and community health services, and to commission hospital care.

Commissioning

PCTs make commissioning decisions. They identify the health needs of the local population and develop a service with healthcare providers to meet those identified needs. This may range from large contracts with healthcare providers to smaller contracts with, for example, voluntary sector providers. PCTs will also commission specialised services (e.g. services for rare cancers) that are only provided in a few centres. This is often achieved by several PCTs working together in specialised commissioning groups.

Practice-based commissioning

Practice-based commissioning means that healthcare professionals and patients may have a greater say in decisions about care providers. This would lead to a greater number of providers giving a wider range of services. It would be more convenient to patients and would also allow more efficient use of resources.

The policy reflects the Government's aims of increasing patient choice and providing alternative routes for patients across primary and secondary care. It is expected that all practices will take part in practice-based commissioning by 2008.

Contracting

PCTs have four options with regard to the provision of primary care services.

1   They can use the General Medical Services (GMS) contract to determine the services that a GP will provide, which allows GP practices some flexibility in the services that they offer.

2   They can use a locally agreed arrangement with practices, namely the Personal Medical Services (PMS) contract. This allows them to offer salaried appointments to GPs. The contract between GPs and PCTs is tailor-made to provide services for identified local needs.

3   They can contract with non-NHS bodies under the alternative provider medical services (APMS) (e.g. voluntary sector or commercial sector independent providers). They can also contract with NHS foundation trusts, NHS trusts or other PCTs to provide primary care services.

4   They can also provide and manage services themselves (PCTMS). This enables them to run hospitals and community health services.

Principles of good primary care

There are five principles of good primary healthcare, namely quality, fairness, accountability, responsiveness and efficiency.

Quality

- All those working in primary care should be knowledgeable about the medical conditions they are likely to encounter as a result of their work, and skilled in both treatment and prevention.

- Professionals should be knowledgeable about the communities with whom they are working.

- When working with other NHS or health-related bodies (e.g. social care services or voluntary services), those working in primary care should be aware of what is happening outside their own field and work towards delivering a service without gain.

- Premises and facilities should be of a good standard, up to date, well maintained and safe.

Fairness

- Services should be consistent in range and quality across the country.

- Primary care should receive an appropriate share of NHS resources.

Accountability

- Services should be reasonably accessible when clinically needed.

- Necessary services should be available to people regardless of age, sex, ethnicity, disability or health status.

Responsiveness

- Services should reflect the needs and choices of those using them.

- Services should reflect the health and needs of the local population.

Efficiency

- Primary care services should be based on evidence of medical effectiveness.

- Primary care resources should be used effectively.

Primary care is the setting in which 90% of patients receive treatment, and advances in modern healthcare mean that more treatments that were once administered in hospitals are now undertaken by primary care providers.

PCTs in some areas are setting up one-stop health centres which bring together GPs, nurses, health visitors, dentists, a pharmacy, a cardiology clinic, X-ray facilities and optometry services under one roof.

Chapter 1 provides detailed information about the following primary care services:

- walk-in centres

- NHS Direct

- NHS Direct Online.

NHS Direct Interactive is an interactive health information service that was developed for digital television. It has many pages of content (in six languages), including a health encyclopaedia, a directory of local NHS trusts, and information on how to use the NHS, as well as advice on diet, health, exercise, etc.

The patient and the receptionist

From the patient's point of view there are no major changes to services, since they are all still available, but they should now be more efficient as they are delivered according to the Patient's Charter. The Patient's Charter is a document that sets out the standard of service to be provided in layman's language.

Receptionists who are arranging access to services will find that procedures depend on local arrangements. Set procedures can only be specified by referring to the local offices of the ambulance service, social or community services. It is advisable for staff responsible for arranging transport to visit ambulance headquarters to see at first hand how requests for transport are processed.

As a result of the growth of the primary healthcare sector, the role of the receptionist, clerical and secretarial staff, both in the hospital and in general practice, is becoming increasingly complex as the changes are effected. No longer do staff merely 'go between' the doctor and patient, but they must now liaise with hospital departments, community and social services. Every few months another department or service moves, changes its name, and its personnel change their function or role. It is important for all staff to understand the difficulties experienced in other sectors of health and social care provision as they cope with the fundamental changes that are going on around them.

Although doctors' surgery staff may have been recognised as part of the primary healthcare team for some time, their importance as key members in providing a communication link is growing with the size of the team and the increased variety of necessary points of contact.

The primary healthcare team

The change of emphasis from institutionalised healthcare provision to management by smaller sections within the services generates a greater need for deliberate integration of the various services so that patients are presented with 'seamless' health and social care.

Staff increasingly become involved in dealing with queries, passing messages, and ensuring that the patients released from long-term institutionalised care, or fresh from surgical procedures, receive the service that they need from the various members of the extended primary healthcare team.

From the 1960s, as health authorities built health centres, accommodation was provided for the community, social and other care services, including chiropody, dental services and dispensaries. This made it easier for doctors and receptionists to communicate with, for example, community staff, because they were likely to meet in the health centre. In the last few years there has been a general move to 'attach' community staff to specific surgeries where the premises are privately owned by the doctors. A message-book is kept in reception so that messages can be picked up easily, and office space is made available.

The benefits of better communication have been supplemented by developing primary healthcare team meetings. These may have a strong clinical flavour, where doctors and health visitors, midwives and social workers discuss the needs of specific patients. Alternatively, meetings where strategies are developed for defining and maintaining management and administration of the team would also include reception and administration staff. It is essential to have a chairperson to control the agenda so that the subject areas are of interest to everyone. Even if meetings are only held monthly, getting together a group of up to 40 people on a regular basis can be extremely difficult. It is important, therefore, to produce brief minutes so that those who are unable to attend can follow up issues with colleagues.

The primary healthcare team in its broadest sense includes doctors, the practice manager, practice nurses, nurse practitioner, reception, secretarial and other administrative staff, health visitors, midwives, community nursing staff, social workers, community psychiatric nurses and any other nursing specialists. Within this team, however, there are other teams (e.g. receptionists, practice nurses, practice secretaries, etc.). Each team should work together for the common good, so it is important for everyone to appreciate the role, purpose and special skills of its members.

Since October 1997, *all* staff working in primary healthcare, including receptionists, secretaries and practice nurses, are eligible to contribute to the NHS Pension Scheme. This development has meant fewer staff changes in the practice team, and has especially encouraged receptionists and secretaries to feel that their skills and experience are recognised and that their employment offers a worthwhile career structure.

The general medical practitioner

The GP is at the centre of primary healthcare. The doctor's surgery represents the entrance to most of the services provided by the NHS, and the GP's responsibility is to maintain the health of patients and their families by treatment, prevention and health education. GPs give personal and continuing care to their patients, and are in a position to build up a relationship of trust. They attend patients both in their consulting room and in their homes. The GP aims to make initial diagnoses of problems presented, to provide treatment as appropriate, or where necessary to refer patients for further professional treatment.

Registrars (trainees)

If the general medical practice is a training practice, the registrar may be part of the medical team. Registrars are fully qualified doctors undergoing the requisite training and gaining expertise in general medical practice.

The practice manager

The practice manager is the person to whom both secretaries and receptionists in general practice are accountable. He or she has a central role in the day-to-day smooth running of the practice to ensure a quality service to the patients. The practice manager is the leader responsible for building, maintaining and co-ordinating the practice team so that the objectives are achieved and tasks completed satisfactorily. He or she also has responsibility for developing and training individuals and helping them to realise their potential. The practice manager is the person to whom secretaries and receptionists will go to discuss any difficulties and problems they experience in the workplace.

The nurse in primary care

The initiative to increase access to primary care, such as walk-in centres, NHS Direct or minor injuries units, has nurses as the initial point of patient contact. Some practices employ nurses to run specialist clinics (e.g. asthma and diabetes clinics), and patients may be offered a direct consultation with the nurse for certain minor conditions. The nurse's role is certainly expanding as they take on more responsibilities. We already have the nurse practitioner role, and a new post of nurse consultant will further enhance the future role of the nurse in primary care.

More nurses are undertaking further training which will enable them to prescribe certain items as stated in the Nurse Prescribers' Formulary or the Extended Formulary in the *British National Formulary* (*see* Chapter 11 for more information).

Community nursing sisters

These used to be known as district nurses because they worked on a geographical basis looking after the nursing needs of patients in their own homes. They are now more often than not attached to a single practice and work with the patients belonging to that practice, or perhaps the patients of two smaller practices. Practice attachment gives them a chance to work more closely in a team with other staff, but has the disadvantage of spreading their work over a very wide area. Occasionally these nurses work in the treatment room of the practice. They are employed by the community health NHS trust, and are fully trained nurses who have gained experience in hospitals before coming to work in the community. They are involved in traditional nursing duties such as treating people who are ill at home with heart failure, acute chest conditions, terminal illness or, increasingly, after early discharge from hospital. These patients may require wound dressings, attention to bowels, prevention of bed sores and so on, and their relatives at home will gain great support from being taught how to help the patient themselves, or just by knowing that someone will be coming in regularly.

Health visitors

The health visitor is a trained nurse with a post-registration qualification, employed by the community health NHS trust, and working mainly as a member of the primary healthcare team. The training of health visitors is rooted in the promotion of health, and they learn to recognise the effects of psychological, social, economic and environmental factors on health. This enables them to fulfil their role in health education and the prevention of disease.

Although health visitors are concerned with all age groups, they have a special responsibility for the under-fives. New-born babies are visited in their own homes, and parents are advised on matters of child health and development. Emphasis is given to the need for immunisation and the value of attending a child health clinic. They are also concerned with other vulnerable groups such as the elderly, the physically and mentally handicapped, single parents, and families under stress. In addition, they may be involved in the provision of health surveillance programmes and research, in which case an age–sex register or other form of database is particularly helpful.

Practice nurses

These nurses form a rapidly growing group of healthcare workers and represent one way in which health services are changing to meet new challenges. They are usually employed by the practice and do most of their work within the treatment room. They are normally fully trained nurses who have gained experience in hospital and other fields before taking up practice work. Practice nurses are employed in traditional work in the treatment room, such as applying dressings, giving injections, syringing ears and removing sutures. The range of their activity is changing to include helping to run health promotion clinics, and assisting with child health surveillance and minor surgery. They are thus often specially trained in the management of chronic illness such as asthma, diabetes and hypertension. Practice nurses are beginning to use some of the tools that were traditionally used only by the doctor, such as ophthalmoscopes, stethoscopes, auriscopes and vaginal speculae. Further important extensions of their work include counselling, listening and reassuring.

Nurse practitioners

Nurse practitioners are nurses with specialist training which allows them to practise independently. In some cases they take on responsibilities similar to those of junior medical staff, and in general practice they may run clinics and assess priorities.

Midwives

Midwives have a central role in the care of pregnant women. They are fully trained nurses who have subsequently completed a prolonged midwifery course. They are employed by the community health NHS trust and they form part of the team with hospital obstetricians, general practitioners and health visitors concerned with antenatal care, antenatal preparation, intrapartum care, delivery, and postpartum care of the mother and infant. They sometimes run antenatal clinics with doctors, and conduct normal deliveries in hospital and occasionally in the home. They are also very much involved in the postpartum care of mothers who are discharged home early after delivery.

Social workers

In about one in five consultations a doctor becomes involved in discussions and advice about personal relationships, work, social benefits, social support or other financial matters. These are important features of primary care, but just as the doctor will want to call upon the special skills of nurses for some problems, so he or she will want to use a social worker's skills for the issues listed above.

For example, if a young single mother is taken ill, the problem extends beyond the immediate care of a sick woman and involves a healthy child as well. If an elderly person living alone has a minor stroke which limits their independence by making it difficult to cook, clean or shop, another type of problem arises that might best be solved by a home help, meals on wheels or laundry services. The social worker will help to assess the need for this service, and to set up these forms of care if they are needed. Again, if family tensions put the wife or children at risk, supervision and counselling may be required, and the problem is most likely to be dealt with by a social worker.

There are some specialised social workers. These include psychiatric social workers, who have an important role in the involuntary admission of the psychiatrically ill and in helping and supporting the long-term sick, such as patients who are schizophrenics, or those with senile dementia who live in the community.

Community psychiatric nurses

Community psychiatric nurses belong to a profession which, although still in its infancy, is of increasing importance. Their role has developed with the trend towards rehabilitating and caring for the mentally infirm in the community. Although they may be employed in psychiatric hospitals, they are largely involved in providing support and treatment in collaboration with general practitioners. They tend to act as independent clinical practitioners themselves, backed by both consultants and general practitioners, with the object of restricting long-term hospital treatment to only the severest cases.

Dentists and dental services

Dentists may also be considered as part of primary care services. Unfortunately, policies on dental services have not been as forthcoming as those for other health sectors. A great deal of publicity has highlighted the problems that many people seeking dental care have encountered (e.g. that it is not available under the NHS, or that NHS dentists are not accepting new patients). As a result, many patients are unwilling or unable to pay for private dental care and are therefore not visiting a dentist on a regular basis.

In 2006 it is expected that an increased budget for primary care dental services will be devolved to PCTs, which will then be able to commission primary dental care. These services will cover surgery salaries and expenses, which will replace the system of payment that was originally set up when the NHS was first established.

The Government is aiming to recruit 1000 more dentists – some from outside the NHS (including some from abroad) – and to provide more undergraduate dental training places in England.

A new contract for dentists is designed to enable them to spend more time with patients, and to give advice about preventive dental care.

Pharmacists

We saw in another section how doctors and pharmacists relate to each other in terms of their activities with prescriptions. Many patients go first to the pharmacist with their complaint, and may never need to see the doctor. Others are advised by the pharmacist that a consultation is necessary. Communication between the two professions is very important.

Optometrists (or ophthalmic opticians)

These are specialist health professionals who test eyes and prescribe lenses to correct sight problems. They are more commonly referred to as 'opticians'. A 'dispensing optician' fits and sells glasses but does not test eyes. An ophthalmic optician specialises in making glasses, testing eyes and prescribing appropriate lenses.

(Detailed information about the above primary care services provision may be found in Chapter 1.)

Home helps

Home helps play a vital role in enabling the elderly to stay in their homes for as long as possible. Their role is to perform those domestic tasks – such as shopping, washing, cleaning and collecting pensions – which the elderly can no longer undertake because of infirmity. They have no clinical responsibility, but their visits provide a friendly and caring link with the outside world. It is usually the social services department of the local authority that organises their work.

Home care teams

We have seen that some teams consist of people employed by the practice, whilst others consist of people employed by the health authorities. There is yet another arm of support, namely voluntary organisations. A particularly good example of this is the hospice which provides care for the terminally ill. Doctors and nurses working in this field, supported mainly by charity, develop a particular expertise and have teams that can visit patients in their own homes by arrangement with the general practitioner.

Other members of the healthcare team

Physiotherapists diagnose and treat patients' difficulties with movement, especially with regard to joints, and assist with rehabilitation after injury. Until recently they worked mainly in hospitals, but an increasing number now work in the community. Physiotherapists will continue with improving the mobility of patients following inpatient hospital procedures and/or as a continuation of rehabilitation after intermediate care services. GPs have direct access to their services.

Social workers can help many patients with problems in non-medical areas of their lives (e.g. living conditions, debts or problems with relationships or child care). The intervention of social workers at an early stage can often help in tackling patients' problems, although these may be closely related to medical conditions for which they consult their doctor. In some areas, GPs employ their own social worker because of the support he or she can give to patients who visit their doctor because they do not know where else to go.

Counsellors may be employed by GPs or attend their surgeries for designated sessions. Early intervention by a counsellor who has time to listen to patients' non-medical problems can help to avert a critical situation.

Dietitians and other care staff advise on the best diet for particular medical conditions. Some health centres and GP practices have a dietitian who attends for designated sessions, working closely with members of the primary healthcare team.

Occupational therapists help patients to resume a normal life after mental or physical illness, through activity-based treatments and the provision of aids to living. They will also assess what alterations are needed to enable elderly or disabled people to continue living at home.

Speech and language therapists help patients who have communication difficulties, especially after stroke or injury. They are trained to diagnose and treat all forms of speech disabilities and disorders of language and articulation in children.

Chiropodists play an important part in helping the elderly (who frequently have debilitating toe and foot problems) to maintain an active role in the community.

Audiometricians do much to help those with hearing disabilities to live a normal and active life.

There is a large variety of other skilled workers who, from time to time, become part of the team. Experts such as chiropodists, dietitians, physiotherapists, clinical psychologists, pharmacists, and so on, may be involved.

The principal skill of clinical psychologists is in the realm of personal development and interpersonal relationships. They can help with behavioural problems in children and teenagers, helping people to cope with life's difficulties, marital problems, and so on.

Other specialist nurses

Specialist nurses working in the community also include the following:

- school nurse

- stoma care nurse

- paediatric nurse

- geriatric nurse

- local authority clinic nurse.

Care trusts

Care trusts allow the integration of health and social care. They commission and provide care within a single NHS organisation.

In some cases the NHS and local authority may establish a joint care trust if both agree that this is the best way to improve health and social care. NHS and local authority functions are delegated to the trust in a voluntary arrangement which enables partners to withdraw if they wish to do so. Care trusts may be based on either an NHS trust or a PCT.

Care trusts tend to focus on specialist health services and services for older people.

Children's trust

In 2004 the Government stated in its Green Paper *Every Child Matters* that it aims to integrate key children's services with a single organisational focus. The trust involves children and their families in putting together an overview of their needs and designing services to meet identified needs. Needs will be met through public, private, community and voluntary service providers.

The first children's commissioner was appointed in March 2005. The role of the English children's commissioner was stated in the Children Act of 2004, which also changed the way in which the NHS works with local authorities to promote the well-being of children. Each authority must set up a children's trust with representatives from education, social services and the primary care trust. In charge of a joint budget, they are meant to commission services in an organised way.

The Act offers flexibility with regard to the form that trusts can take. For example, some will be fully integrated bodies like NHS care trusts, pooling staff and taking responsibility for all children's services. Others will be more specialised and take the form of regular board meetings at which representatives of the key partners will decide how to spend funds.

Both the children's commissioner for England and the children's trust must bear in mind the following key outcomes stated in the Children Act:

- physical and mental health and emotional well-being

- protection from harm and neglect

- education, training and recreation

- the contribution made by children to society

- social and economic well-being.

Managed clinical networks

Joint working between the NHS and local authorities is becoming increasingly important, but sometimes it can be difficult to achieve.

Clinical networks are partnerships of all the organisations and professionals that are involved in commissioning, planning, and providing a service in a geographical area. They have the potential to break down barriers between primary, secondary and tertiary care and between health and social care, and to involve the voluntary sector and local authorities.

Local strategic partnerships (LSPs)

Local strategic partnerships are intended to bring together different parts of the public and private sectors as well as the community and voluntary sectors. They enable decisions to be taken at a community level. The NHS plays an important part in LSPs by improving health and reducing health inequalities.

Public health

Public health is concerned with improving the population's health rather than with treating the diseases of individual patients. One definition of public health, devised by the former Chief Medical Officer, is 'the science and art of preventing disease, prolonging life, and promoting health through the organised efforts of society'. It will be noted from the above text that this is best achieved by collaboration, as many of the aims of public health can only be achieved by partnerships between the Government, the NHS, local authorities and the private and voluntary sectors. Public health professionals monitor the health status of the community, identify needs, develop programmes to reduce risk, and screen for early disease (e.g. regular mammography services and the proposed programme to screen for early signs of bowel cancer). They also control communicable disease, promote health, and plan and evaluate healthcare provision.

The Government's White Paper *Choosing Health*, which was published in 2004, is based on the principle that the NHS should improve health and prevent disease, rather than only providing treatment and care for those who are already ill. It states that people should make their own choices about their lifestyle and, of course, about their health. These should be informed choices about the available services.

This approach to public health is based on the following principles:

- informed choices – people want to be able to make their own decisions about choices that affect their health, and to have good-quality information to help them to do so

- personalisation – support must be tailored to individuals

- working together – progress depends on effective partnerships across communities.

The Government asked Derek Wanless (following his earlier report on NHS resources in the future) to look at the prevention of ill health. His subsequent report (published in 2004) stated that urgent and concerted action was needed at all levels to move away from 'a national sickness service which treats disease to a national health service which focuses on preventing it'.

The public health workforce consists of people from a range of professional disciplines, who are working in one of three categories:

1 *health improvement and reducing inequalities* – teachers, local business leaders, government staff and voluntary sector personnel, as well as doctors and other healthcare professionals

2 *public health practice* – health visitors, environmental health officers and those who use research information, public health science or health promotion skills

3   *public health consultants and specialists* – people who work at a senior
    management level of scientific expertise.

Reducing health inequalities is a Government priority. Action to break the
cycle of deprivation (unemployment and poor housing are major causes of
ill health) and its impact on health is an important issue. Joint working
partnerships, networking, shared funding and shared resources are
crucial at all levels – national, regional and local.

Health promotion

Approximately 25 years ago, health education was a new field seeking to
make information about health matters available to anyone who wanted
it. Health education councils generated literature and visited surgeries,
schools and hospitals to circulate information. In the last five years there
has been an increase in health promotion in doctors' surgeries which has
supplemented health education. Every opportunity is taken to draw
attention to health issues, advise individuals to bring them to a point of
decision about making changes in their lifestyle, and then give out
literature to educate further on how and why to make such changes.
Health promotion draws attention to the need to change, and educates
sufficiently to enable a patient to make an informed choice to change.
Support during the change process and further education with literature
must then follow. The terms 'education' and 'promotion' refer to different
aspects, but to effect change in patient behaviour the two must work hand
in hand.

General practitioners and healthcare providers have been required to
extend their services into promotion of health, as well as looking after the
sick. Surgeries have implemented health promotion clinics, such as well-
man and well-woman clinics, where patients are asked for details of their
lifestyle and given advice on how they might prevent ill health by changes
to their diet, drinking habits, smoking habits, exercise levels and so on.
Where needs such as help in giving up smoking are identified, specific
clinics are then provided in some surgeries, so that patients benefit from
peer group support.

However, all members of the primary healthcare team, including
receptionists and secretaries, are now required to be far more aware of
promoting health. Just as one would find it difficult to accept advice from
an obviously overweight practice nurse advising that one must lose at
least two stones in weight in the next six months, it is important that
healthcare staff present a healthy image – which may include not being
seen smoking – to back up the message that the practitioners and other
health professionals give out daily.

Patient waiting-areas should be used to the full to promote health, with
good-quality notices tidily displayed on notice-boards, and to educate by

leaflets that are available for patients to read while they are waiting, or to take home with them. It may be the practice nurse's responsibility to maintain notice-boards and supplies of leaflets, but it is important that receptionists keep their eyes open and draw the nurse's attention to notice-boards that are looking unkempt or leaflet supplies that are running low.

General practices have also found that 'open days' are an excellent opportunity to give out health promotion messages, when patients are invited into the surgery, perhaps on a Saturday afternoon, to have blood pressure and cholesterol checks, and so on.

The educational aspect is supported by most schools, which ask health visitors and social workers to speak to children and answer questions about what they can do to help themselves. Schools may also invite specific organisations, such as ASH (anti-smoking), substance abuse or local AIDS charities, to educate students about their particular area of expertise.

Since there are 1001 sources of educational information, the role of staff is to be aware of where materials can be obtained for a wide range of subjects, so that literature can be accessed without undue delay. Where literature is not available free of charge, details of costs might be kept on record together with the addresses and contact numbers.

The range of effects on individual lives that might contribute to ill health makes it impossible to generalise about how effective any one particular message might have been. However, research to date shows that eating 'healthily', taking regular exercise and practising moderation in alcohol intake, together with refraining from smoking, all contribute to remaining healthier for longer. Where large-scale health promotion in partnership with health education has been government sponsored, as in Finland, treatment for and deaths from heart disease have been reduced.

Therefore it is part of the role of the receptionist to support initiatives to promote better health, not only by being aware of the advice given out by doctors and health professionals, but also by advising patients to attend health promotion clinics or events put on by the surgery, and by themselves presenting a healthy image to patients.

Local authority social services

Major local authorities have a social services committee, with an appointed director in charge of its social services department, who co-ordinates and administers the authority's social services.

Secretaries and receptionists will inevitably be asked by patients for information and advice about social services provision, and should have the relevant information readily available to enable them to deal with such queries in a helpful, positive way.

Structure and social services provided

The organisation of the social services department will vary from one area to another, but there are usually at least seven main sections of a social services department:

- residential services

- intermediate care services

- fieldwork services

- respite care services

- provision of training facilities

- hospital social work

- administration.

The following is a summary of the services provided by social services committees:

- *care of the elderly* – this includes both fieldwork services carried out within the community and residential care

- *care of the physically handicapped* – this includes blind, deaf, dumb, hearing difficulties, spastic, epileptic, paraplegics and other disabled people

- *social work advice to the homeless* – this includes provision of permanent accommodation, care of homeless families, advice and help on prevention of homelessness, and bed-and-breakfast accommodation.

Note: Those who are homeless are 'priority'. 'Priority' means anyone who has one or more children living with them, anyone who is made homeless (e.g. by fire or flood), any household which includes one or more people who are elderly or mentally/physically handicapped, or suffer from physical disability, battered wives, and pregnant women. The homeless are also divided into those made *homeless by chance* and those made *homeless intentionally*.

- *Child care services* – child care protection/supervision; acceptance of parental responsibility for children committed into care of the local authority; control of residential units; admission units; reception centres; residential nurseries; children's homes; community homes with education on the premises and classifying homes; adoption services; child abuse/prevention of child abuse services.

- *Social work and family casework dealing with mental disorder* – provision of social workers; adult training centres; workshops; residential accommodation (hostels).

- *Day care for children under five years of age* – provision of day nurseries, supervision of private nurseries and childminders.

- *Provision of home carers.*

- *Care of unsupported mothers* – including residential care.

- *Hospital social workers* – provision of social work services for hospital patients.

- *Work in the field of alcohol and drug abuse.*

It will have been noted that social services offer a wide range of services for people who are at risk or who have a high level of need, and aim to protect and support vulnerable people by helping them to live independently.

Assessment

An assessment of needs is conducted by a member of specialist staff in the home, in hospital, or in the social services office. The assessment gives the person concerned the opportunity to discuss their needs.

Social work teams

A team of area social workers undertakes all of the casework for family and clients, so that problems can be considered as a whole, thus leading to family social services, helping all kinds of social problems in the family. Teams are composed of specialist social workers (e.g. specialists in child care, mental illness or handicap, physical handicap, and care of the elderly). It is the area social work team which usually co-ordinates the allocation of the following:

- home carers

- meals on wheels

- day-nursery places

- vacancies in residential homes for the elderly

- residential accommodation for children.

Health and social services liaison

Social services work in close liaison with the local health authority to provide support and help in the community to patients recently discharged from hospital, or suffering from a disabling condition. The necessary adaptations, gadgets and aids for these people that are vital for their rehabilitation are supplied by the occupational therapy section of the social services department.

A community physician who is a specialist in community medicine is responsible for liaison between health and social services. Social workers now visit medical practices and health centres, where they meet general practitioners, health visitors, community nurses and school nurses working from these centres.

Community care

Social services departments will continue to work closely with health authorities to plan and provide 'care packages' to give the support that people need to help in their daily lives, and may be available from local government and health authorities. It involves both social and healthcare, and the Government will continue to encourage purchasers and providers to work with local authority partners to ensure that arrangements for community care work effectively. One of the major aims of community care is to enable people to maximise their independence by living in their own home for as long as possible, and when this is no longer practicable, to find them a home-like place to live.

Mental health services are provided as part of primary and secondary care, with responsibility divided between the NHS, social services and the voluntary sector. PCTs are responsible for commissioning all mental health services, or may even provide these services in partnership with a specialist provider. This will bring services closer to users, reflect local problems and encourage partnership between health and social care. Specialist mental health trusts provide inpatient care as well as rehabilitation services, residential care centres, day centres and drop-in centres.

The majority of patients who are experiencing mental health problems use only primary care services.

Community mental health team (CMHT)

CMHTs (also known as primary care liaison teams) support people with mental health problems. They assess and monitor mental health needs by using either the Care Programme Approach or care management. Patients who are seen by CMHTs have their need for treatment assessed and a care plan is drawn up. A named mental health worker co-ordinates their care and reviews them on a regular basis.

The aim of CMHTs is to provide continuity of care, ensuring appropriate care for people with serious mental disorders.

Members of the CMHT include the following:

- community psychiatric nurses

- social workers

- psychologists

- doctors

- occupational therapists

- support workers.

Care Programme Approach

The Care Programme Approach is the way in which specialist mental health services are delivered to those who need them, and patients can expect the following:

- an assessment of their health and social care needs

- a written plan to meet those needs

- to be involved in drawing up their care plan

- a regular review of their care plan

- to have a named mental health worker (a care co-ordinator or key-worker) who is responsible for the patient's care under the Care Programme Approach.

New rights for carers

From 1 April 1996, carers were given new rights under a new law called the Carers Recognition and Services Act (otherwise known as the Carers Act). This Act entitles carers to an assessment in their own right. Social services departments will have to listen to carers, record their views and take into account the result of the carer's assessment when they decide what services to bring to the person who is being cared for. The Carers Act states that carers are people who look after and support sick, elderly and disabled relatives and friends, providing a substantial amount of care on a regular basis.

Summary

The foregoing account is intended to stress the importance to secretaries and receptionists of having sources of information at their fingertips so that they are able to answer, with knowledge and understanding, the numerous and diverse questions that will be put to them by patients and their relatives.

At the time of writing, many changes are taking place in both primary care and social care of patients, often in partnership with a specialist provider. As a result, staff should ensure that they have an understanding of the changes taking place so that they are able to answer all of the queries that may be put to them.

Useful websites

www.bma.org.uk/gpcontract
www.dh.gov.uk/policyandguidance

13

Audit, health economics and ensuring quality for the medical receptionist and secretary

Introduction

Receptionists and secretaries working in the healthcare field will no doubt be aware of the emergence of new concepts and buzzwords or phrases for a wide variety of initiatives and processes, all aimed at benefiting the patient. The most important of these issues are considered to give the reader an underpinning knowledge and understanding of concepts that are influencing the NHS today.

As receptionists and secretaries in the NHS or other healthcare organisations, you should remember that the way in which you work must always be of the highest standard. Errors have arisen in the past which may have put a patient's life in danger, when computer data have been carelessly keyed by a member of staff, or when a word has been mistyped (e.g. the words 'hypotension' and 'hypertension' are very similar, but have different meanings). Other examples of transcription mistakes have been reported (e.g. a 'below-knee amputation' was transcribed as 'baloney amputation' and 'Eustachian tube malfunction' was transcribed as 'Euston station tube malfunction'). Some of these errors may be amusing, but remember that a misunderstanding of drug quantities could cause real problems (e.g. 15 mg being mistaken for 50 mg). Accuracy of information is of prime importance at all times, whether you are taking down messages over the telephone, typing a patient's report or inputting data.

Figure 13.1

STEPS IN AUDIT

1 Define
criteria and standards

4 Identify
need for change

2 Collect
data on performance

3 Assess
performance against criteria and standards

Audit

Receptionists and secretaries in their day-to-day activities can consider what they do and if they can do it better to provide a quality service to patients. This may include the following:

1 identifying or defining criteria and standards in order to answer the question 'What are we doing/trying to achieve for our patients?'
2 collecting data on current performance (i.e. the care and/or service given and its effects on patients). Are patients satisfied?
3 assessing performance against criteria to determine whether standards have been met and objectives achieved
4 identifying the need for change or improvement in patient care.

The importance of audit

Decision making can only be truly effective when it is based on accurate record keeping and information about various activities. For example, receptionists may be asked to keep records of the numbers of patients seen at the surgery or in the hospital clinic. This is important in decision making to improve the quality of care or service to patients:

• to introduce a new clinic

• to extend the length of the surgery or clinic

- to check that the current consultation system is working satisfactorily in the best interests of both doctors and patients

- to increase staffing levels.

Secretaries and receptionists may feel that the information or statistics which are kept to help decision making are never-ending, but it must be remembered that the conclusions drawn may affect all members of the team and foster a feeling of team spirit and involvement. This in turn will create a professional and caring team that plays an important part in the delivery of a high standard of service and healthcare.

Health economics and cost-effective medicine

Although it is appreciated that readers of this book are unlikely to become involved in these processes, an insight will provide an understanding of some of the dominant political and economic issues facing the NHS and healthcare today. The UK, like many other nations, has experienced a rapid increase in healthcare expenditure, and with it health economics.

Health economics

Economics is concerned with the way in which people earn their living and how they spend their earnings, particularly on goods and services. Health economics is defined as the way in which resources are allocated to health-related issues and the increasing cost of providing a quality healthcare system. As expenditure on healthcare has increased dramatically over the past 30 years, it is not surprising that health economics has emerged as a speciality in its own right and has shown a rapid expansion.

Economics can be divided into two main areas:

- macroeconomics

- microeconomics.

Macroeconomics is concerned with the functioning of the whole economy. Microeconomics is concerned with the functioning of individual parts of the economic system (e.g. the price of a particular product or service, or the behaviour of an individual organisation/institution, and so on). Healthcare is part of the microeconomic system concerned with the effects of expenditure in supplying the needs and demands made upon it. It focuses on the choices made by individuals within the health system.

Evidence-based and cost-effective medicine

The philosophy of evidence-based medicine encourages the medical profession to base the practice of medicine on proven effective treatments or services which are of benefit to, and in the best interests of, patients, yet which at the same time consider the cost-effectiveness of such treatment. It is based on evidence resulting from medical research, comparisons and outcomes of clinical audit. Consideration is given to the cost of providing such treatment, the availability of funds and the quality of patient care.

A new performance framework for the NHS and social care came into effect in April 2005, which sets out the level of quality that all organisations which provide NHS care and those working in the private and voluntary sectors will be expected to meet or aspire to.

The Healthcare Commission has devised a new system for assessing the performance of NHS organisations which is based on the core and development standards framework. It examines the following two areas:

1   getting the basics right, including core standards, national targets, financial position and management, value for money and findings from other regulatory bodies

2   making and sustaining progress, including the following national priorities in the Department of Health's public service agreement:

    – improve the health of the population

    – improve the health of people with long-term conditions

    – improve access to services

    – improve the experience of the patient and the user.

Private Finance Initiative

The Private Finance Initiative (PFI), which was first announced in the 1992 Budget, is intended to harness private-sector management expertise and efficiency in delivering public services. In the NHS it has included the building and servicing of new district general hospital facilities as well as a range of smaller projects.

The PFI involves a public–private partnership between an NHS organisation and a private-sector consortium that makes available private capital for health service projects. All major NHS capital projects are expected to consider whether the PFI could represent a cost-effective solution.

For example, some trusts have been able to replace ageing X-ray equipment through a PFI contract, and as a result now have state-of-the-art scanning equipment in their imaging department. It has been suggested that private contractors may play a key role in the new generation of 'fast-track' treatment centres through PFI-style contracts.

The Department of Health has standardised contracts with PFI consortia – specially created companies which negotiate contracts on behalf of building and finance managers.

The scheme enables the NHS to harness private-sector expertise, allowing NHS management to concentrate on delivering cost-effective clinical services and ultimately providing better value for money.

Plans to redevelop existing hospitals by providing updated facilities and more sophisticated diagnostic equipment are going ahead, with finance being made available through the public–private partnership (PPP) initiative.

Clinical governance

Clinical governance is a statutory duty aimed at 'ensuring that all NHS organisations have in place proper processes for continuously monitoring and improving clinical audit'. Clinicians and managers will be expected to understand their individual and collective responsibilities for assuring accountability for the quality of patient healthcare, and take on a legal responsibility for standards of health service treatment.

One tool of clinical governance designed to improve the quality of medical care might be clinical audit, which evaluates the results and effectiveness of treatment. In this way it is possible to identify improvements, or the need for them, which have occurred in medical practice over a period of time, and to identify medical standards and guidelines based on research evidence. Clinical governance means that every healthcare professional should be responsible and accountable for his or her own personal standards of practice.

National Institute for Clinical Excellence (NICE)

NICE is a special health authority that was set up in 1999. It provides guidance for professionals, managers, patients and carers on decisions about treatment and healthcare, which covers the following:

- clinical guidelines

- technology appraisals

- the use of new surgical or other interventional procedures.

National Clinical Assessment Service (NCAS)

The NCAS is responsible to the National Patient Safety Agency and provides a central point of contact when concerns about an individual doctor's or dentist's performance are raised.

National Service Frameworks (NSFs)

NSFs are evidence-based programmes that set quality standards and help to establish clear national standards to improve quality, reduce unacceptable variations in the standards of care and treatment, and generally promote collaboration between organisations and contribute to improving public health.

It is usual for only one NSF to be released each year. The programme began in 1998 and now covers the following areas:

- mental health (September 1999)

- coronary heart disease (March 2000)

- cancer (September 2000)

- older people (March 2001)

- diabetes – standards (December 2001) and delivery strategy (January 2003)

- renal services – Part One (January 2001) and Part Two (February 2005)

- children, young people and maternity services (September 2004)

- long-term conditions (March 2005).

Patient surveys

National patient surveys

The Healthcare Commission is responsible for conducting national survey programmes. In order to deliver an improved service, the NHS has to know people's needs and expectations. These surveys have three important aims:

1   to provide feedback for local quality improvement

2   to assess users' experience

3   to monitor patients' experience on a national basis.

In 2004 the Healthcare Commission conducted five national survey programmes covering the following areas:

- adult inpatients
- young patients
- primary care
- mental health
- ambulance services.

Local patient surveys

A requirement of the NHS Plan is for each trust to obtain feedback from its own patients about their experiences of care. Receptionists and secretaries may be involved in obtaining relevant feedback from patients. These surveys have the following aims:

- to track changes in patients' experience at trusts, year on year
- to provide information for local quality improvement initiatives
- to inform each trust's performance.

Trusts are able to obtain support and help in conducting these surveys from the NHS Patient Survey Programme Advice Centre (www.nhssurveys.org).

Summary

Many initiatives designed to ensure the accountability and quality of patient care and efficient medical practice have been introduced in recent years. The Healthcare Commission has replaced the Commission for Health Improvement and is responsible for promoting quality standards and keeping a watchful eye on both the NHS and private healthcare service activity.

It concentrates on quality issues and ensures that mechanisms for improving the quality of service are proving to be efficient and effective.

Conclusion

Although they are not directly involved in the concepts discussed in this chapter, receptionists and secretaries form an integral part of a healthcare team which is committed to providing patients with high-quality and cost-effective care. It is important to remember that every member of the team is involved in collecting the data necessary to assess the quality of care, and if change is indicated as an outcome of audit, then teamwork is essential to achieving the wider context of quality in healthcare provision.

Throughout this book you will have noticed other areas of audit and emphasis on issues which are aimed at improving the quality of patient care throughout the NHS and the private and voluntary sectors. This is an extremely important aspect of your work.

14

Training and development

Introduction

Training and development should also be considered as ways of improving your personal effectiveness. Before we consider this in more detail, it is important to distinguish between the following:

- training
- education
- development.

Training is a systematic process for developing the skills, knowledge and attitudes applied to a specific type of work. It is the process of bringing a person to an agreed standard of competence by practice or instruction.

Education is the process of acquiring background knowledge and skills. It does not have to be specific to a particular area of work.

Development is a course of action which enables individuals to realise their potential for growth and promotion in an organisation.

Well-trained receptionists and secretaries are valued members of the work team, and are better able to understand, appreciate and contribute to the smooth running of the medical practice or hospital department.

Excellent training courses are available, and may be provided as in-house training in the work environment, or by external training providers (e.g. health authorities and colleges of further education) (*see* Appendix 3). Training courses leading to a recognised qualification may necessitate attendance at a college on a day release basis, or may be provided as short training courses which take place in the evening.

Why train?

The reasons for training staff are varied, but generally they will fall into one of the following categories:

1 induction needs of new staff:
   • introduction to the practice, the practice team and practice objectives
   • information about the workplace and conditions of employment
   • initial job training
2 to help staff to improve their performance at work:
   • where staff need further training to enable them to do their job at the required level of competence
3 further job training:
   • to give fuller job-related training in specific areas/tasks
4 personal development:
   • training provided where staff wish to develop their career (e.g. by attending a course to gain a professional qualification)
5 retraining:
   • where the nature of the job changes and retraining is necessary to enable the individual to carry out the new work competently
6 policy implementation:
   • staff training may be necessary to ensure that national criteria are implemented
7 response to organisational change:
   • training is necessary where staff are required to respond to changes that affect their jobs (e.g. introduction of new technology, improving teamwork, teambuilding, etc.).

Training strategies

There are six main training strategies that are appropriate to the needs of receptionists and secretaries:

• *on-the-job* – may be carried out by the individual's immediate supervisor in the workplace

- *planned organisational experience* – in-house training, such as a special project to investigate a problem (e.g. appointments system not working well) and make recommendations for improvement

- *in-house courses* – suitable for short-term training needs to target a specific area, and carried out by the individual's immediate supervisor or an external trainer

- *off-the-job (external courses)* – regular attendance at a college or training centre offering specific courses/qualifications

- *open/distance learning* – training courses designed to give greater flexibility and suitable where regular attendance is impractical

- *on-line learning* – more and more educational providers are not only providing traditional tutorial support for open and distance learning training courses, but are also offering on-line and web-based support as well as opportunities to join in discussions with tutors and other students.

Self-development

Self-development is the development of yourself, by yourself, through a deliberate process of learning from experience. This definition assumes that you need to organise it for yourself, rather than expect other people to be responsible for your development. If you do not take responsibility for your own development, who else will? The door to development is locked – you are the keyholder!

Your manager is responsible for providing you with development opportunities, but it is always up to the individual to take the opportunities on offer and make something of them.

The NHS Plan

The NHS Plan confirms the need for employers to provide training opportunities for individual members of staff to further their careers. The deadline of April 2001 was stated for employers to organise a training and development plan for all of their staff which should be linked to appraisal systems.

The NHS Plan has promised an individual leaning account (ILA) for all staff who do not have a professional qualification, or training, to NVQ Level 2 or 3. Both NVQs and ILA offer a means of assuring quality standards in the workplace. ILAs have been developed by the Department of Education and Employment and provide the opportunity for learning about many aspects of healthcare.

NHS staff are able to apply for a place on this scheme.

National Vocational Qualifications (NVQs)

National Vocational Qualifications (NVQs) were introduced in order to replace the varied range of occupational qualifications with an assessed set of standards, which are created by national training and employer-led organisations. These organisations represent an occupational or industrial sector.

NVQs provide a flexible means of obtaining a qualification. There is virtually no time limit, and there are no examinations. They are composed of units which describe the skills and knowledge which are necessary to carry out a job efficiently, and they may be described as a statement of performance.

More and more training and development programmes and learning materials are designed to provide the underpinning knowledge and understanding which facilitate the achievement of competence towards NVQs (SNVQs in Scotland).

NVQs (and SNVQs) are based on what people need to be able to do in order to carry out their jobs competently. They are work-based competences, which are assessed in the workplace. The qualifications are based on completion of units and elements and achievement of stated standards of performance criteria.

NVQs (and SNVQs) are assessed on the production of evidence of achievement, and secretaries and receptionists who wish to achieve NVQs (or SNVQs) should gather evidence in the form of a 'portfolio'. A portfolio is a collection of evidence demonstrating competence which can be based on previous as well as current learning.

The system is accredited by the Qualifications Curriculum Authority (QCA), which was set up in 1997 to regulate all external qualifications in England, Wales, Northern Ireland and Scotland.

All awarding bodies (e.g. the RSA Examinations Board) that wish to accredit national qualifications must apply to the QCA to achieve nationally accredited awarding body status.

NHS staff without a professional qualification are eligible to apply for a place on this scheme. All such staff will have access to an ILA of £150 or dedicated training to NVQ (Level 2 or 3). As a result of this investment, it is anticipated that the NHS will better use its staff, including healthcare assistants, pharmacy technicians, operating department practitioners and administrative staff, thus providing an improved standard of patient care.

A national framework is in place to implement this scheme, helping employers to make work-related training available to their staff.

The NHS University (NHSU)

The NHSU was launched in December 2003, with the aim of putting learning at the heart of the health service and offering training to more than 25 000 NHS employees. It ceased to exist as an independent body in July 2005. The NHSU has now been merged with the Modernisation Agency and the NHS Leadership Centre to form the NHS Institute for Learning, Skills and Innovation (NILSI). Some of the NHSU's work will be continued by NILSI, while other projects will be transferred or discontinued.

NILSI's role will be to help to disseminate and commercialise innovative work in the NHS healthcare industry. It will produce support materials to help individuals, teams and organisations.

Career structure

Secretaries and receptionists working in the field of healthcare are in a position, with their experience and further training, to progress to achieve the position of senior secretary or receptionist, and could well progress further to a supervisory or management role within the organisation.

An opportunity to discuss career development and any training needs could be identified at your annual performance appraisal, and a personal development plan arranged.

Summary

Training and development contribute to your personal effectiveness as a medical secretary or receptionist, and also to being a more effective and highly valued member of the work team.

There are several professional organisations that offer recognised qualifications. Your practice manager, training manager or your local college will be able to provide you with further information.

(*See* Appendix 3 for further information about training providers and courses.)

15

Complementary medicine

Introduction

This chapter on complementary medicine/therapy is included because the term is recognised by the public and acknowledged by the medical profession. A term that was used in a published report by the British Medical Association in 1933 was 'non-conventional therapy'. Treatments which can be used alongside conventional Western, science-based medical care are best described as 'complementary' and are in some instances provided by the NHS. On the other hand 'alternative therapies' replace conventional treatments.

Medical receptionists and secretaries working either for the NHS or in private practice or hospital may be involved in dealing with patients' enquiries about such provision, with the prior approval of the healthcare professionals involved, of course. This chapter aims to give the reader an outline of non-conventional therapies (*see* Appendix 13 for a list of useful addresses), and to provide an overview of some which are practised in the UK.

Acupuncture

This traditional 4000-year-old Chinese healing system came to Europe in the nineteenth century.

Medical or Western acupuncture is based on traditional Chinese medicine, and is practised by doctors on the medical register. It is a touch technique based on the theory of body meridian lines, or lines of energy. Needles are inserted along the meridians in order to balance the body's *yin* and *yang* energy flows and thereby restore or promote the healing forces of the body. Medical or Western acupuncture is also used to achieve anaesthesia. Doctors, physiotherapists and nurses must successfully undertake a two-year course of postgraduate study in order to be registered to practise acupuncture.

Alexander technique

The Alexander technique was developed in the 1890s by an Australian actor whose breathing problems affected his career. It is a method of postural correction and re-education in which people are taught to stand and move efficiently. It teaches a more natural way of moving and of supporting one's weight, and a way of monitoring how to do this. It is not a direct treatment or a cure for a specific illness, but rather an educational method to improve a person's overall functioning.

The Society of Teachers of the Alexander Technique supervises training and maintains a code of ethics and a register of teachers.

Aromatherapy

Aromatherapy originated in the Middle East and was introduced to Europe by the Romans. It is a touch technique based on the healing properties of essential plant oils. Holistic aromatherapy uses massage and essential oils to treat emotional and physical problems. Aromatherapy is not a regulated therapy, and unqualified individuals may set up as practitioners. However, an Aromatherapy Council was set up in 1991 with the aim of setting standards with 50 hours of clinical training followed by an examination. Success in the latter would give entry to the Register of Qualified Aromatherapists.

Chiropractic

Chiropractic was developed by a Canadian osteopath to treat musculo skeletal disorders and their effect on the nervous system by manipulation and soft tissue massage. Therapists use spinal X-rays for the diagnosis of mechanical problems. Appropriate exercises and postural advice are given. Qualification is by a five-year full-time degree course followed by one year in a British Chiropractic Association clinic, after which an honorary doctorate of chiropractic is obtained.

Homeopathy

Homeopathy is yet another ancient treatment dating back to the fourth century BC, when Hippocrates suggested that treatment with something that mimics illness might cure it. Patients in Europe have been treated by this principle since the late eighteenth century, and homeopathy is now well established in the UK, with hundreds of medically qualified doctors registered as homeopaths.

Treatment consists of the administration of greatly diluted forms of natural substances that in a healthy person would produce symptoms similar to those which the medicine is prescribed to treat.

The Statutory Faculty of Homeopathy trains and registers medical practitioners in homeopathy.

Hydrotherapy

Although hydrotherapy cannot be referred to as *complementary* medicine, as it is an orthodox treatment practised by appropriately qualified chartered physiotherapists, it is becoming increasingly recognised as an effective therapy. Hydrotherapy consists of physiotherapy exercises and treatment in a warm, shallow pool heated to approximately 35°C. The warmth of the water and the natural buoyancy supporting the limbs enable movements to be carried out which could not normally be performed on dry land.

Hydrotherapy also improves the circulation, relieves pain and stiffness, and improves mobility and posture. It is used mainly in the effective treatment of many locomotor disorders, including rheumatic and arthritic conditions, in addition to pre- and postoperative rehabilitation of joint replacement, spinal surgery, fractures and sports injuries. Hydrotherapy is practised by a registered physiotherapist who has undertaken a postgraduate course in hydrotherapy.

Hypnotherapy

This therapy was first used by the Greeks to treat problems such as anxiety and hysteria. An eighteenth-century Austrian physician, Franz Mesmer, successfully treated people by putting them into a trance. Subsequently, a French physician, Ambrose Lebeaut, developed the technique of hypnosis.

In hypnotherapy, the patient is made to relax with the use of hypnosis. The therapy is aimed at reducing pain, bringing about changes in mental state and making suggestions for relieving symptoms.

Many doctors, dentists and psychologists are clinically trained in hypnotherapy, but anyone can set up as a hypnotherapist, as there is no regulatory body. The duration of training may vary from one or two days to several months. The National School of Hypnotherapy and Psycho-therapy offers training courses.

Osteopathy

Osteopathy was founded in the nineteenth century by an American who was both a doctor and an engineer, and the technique arrived in the UK at the beginning of the twentieth century. The first school of osteopathy was established in 1917 in London.

Osteopathy is a system of diagnosis and healing that aims to improve the functioning of the body through its structure. It works primarily through articulation and mobilisation of the musculoskeletal system (the bones and soft tissues of the body) in order to influence the nerve supply, the blood supply, the fluid systems and the energy systems of the body and maximise the body's self-healing ability. Although generally associated with the treatment of back pain and bone disorders, osteopathy is now used to relieve a wide variety of ailments, including digestive, respiratory and circulatory problems, neck pain, joint pain and mobility problems.

Practitioners use mainly gentle manual manipulative methods to restore and maintain biomechanical function.

Osteopathy was the first complementary therapy to be statutorily regulated in the UK. The Osteopaths Act of 1993 protects patients from untrained practitioners. Since 1999, all osteopaths have had to be registered with the General Osteopathic Council which holds a list of professional requirements, recognised qualifications and compulsory preregistration training.

Reflexology

Over 5000 years ago, hand and foot massage was practised in China and India. In the nineteenth century an American surgeon noticed that when pressure was applied to certain areas of the hand and foot, partial anaesthesia to the nose and throat was produced, allowing minor surgery to be performed. This concept was developed and introduced to the UK. Reflexology consists of compression and massage techniques using reflex areas of the feet and hands, and is designed to stimulate the blood supply and nerves, thus relieving tension. It may also be used as an indicator of possible problems in various parts of the body.

The Association of Reflexologists gives accreditation to courses in the UK, and the British Reflexology Association is a representative professional organisation. Both organisations have codes of practice and ethics, as well as holding lists of accredited therapists.

Summary

An overview of the most widely used forms of complementary medicine has been given, although it is appreciated that other non-conventional therapies have been found to have a beneficial effect. These include the following:

- herbalism

- massage (touch)

- tai chi (oriental, self-help, postural)

- yoga (oriental, self-help, postural).

Further reading and reference books

Medical secretaries and receptionists should know the sources from which information can be obtained. The following list will be of value.

Medical reference

*   *Medical Dictionary – Dorland's Pocket Medical Dictionary*
    Pocket Medical Dictionary, Churchill Livingstone.

*   *The Medical Directory* – consists of two volumes containing a directory of all qualified medical practitioners, with addresses, qualifications and posts held. Information about hospitals is also included. There will usually be a recent copy at your place of employment.

*   *First Aid Manual* – the authorised manual of St John's Ambulance Association, St Andrew's Ambulance Association and the British Red Cross Society.

*   *British National Formulary* – this contains accurate information about all proprietary drugs.

*   *MIMS* – a monthly publication listing all proprietary drugs and their uses.

General reference

English

*   *The Concise Oxford Dictionary* or *Chambers Dictionary*.

*   Fowler's *Modern English Usage* – a helpful reference book for problems relating to English usage and grammar.

*   Roget's *Thesaurus of English Words and Phrases* – this book lists words according to their meaning.

Information about correct forms of address will assist the secretary in ascertaining decorations, honours and qualifications, and placing them in the correct sequence. For example:

- Black's *Titles and Forms of Address*
- Debrett's *Peerage and Baronetage*
- *Who's Who*.

Travel information/guides

The secretary may find the following helpful, but up-to-date information should always be obtained from appropriate sources:

- railway and airways guides
- railway timetables
- Automobile Association (AA) and Royal Automobile Club (RAC) handbooks – these give useful information for motorists and details of hotels, etc.

Addresses and telephone numbers

Reference can be made to telephone directories and *Yellow Pages* for addresses and telephone numbers and listings of names under professions or trades.

The Post Office Directory can be used for detailed information of streets and occupiers of each house/shop, etc.

General

The following are useful:

- *Whitaker's Almanac*
- *Guide to your Local Social Services Provision*
- *Post Office Guide*
- *Voluntary Services Guide*
- *Pear's Cyclopaedia*.

Further reading

- Bryans W (2004) *Managing in Health and Social Care: essential checklists for frontline staff*. Radcliffe Publishing Ltd, Oxford.
- Bryans W (2005) *Resource Management in Health and Social Care: essential checklists*. Radcliffe Publishing Ltd, Oxford.
- Carr S (2002) *Tackling NHS Jargon: getting the message across*. Radcliffe Medical Press, Oxford.
- Chambers R (2005) *Career Planning for Everyone in the NHS: the toolkit*. Radcliffe Publishing Ltd, Oxford.
- Chambers R, Boath E and Rogers D (2004) *Clinical Effectiveness and Clinical Governance Made Easy* (3e) Radcliffe Publishing Ltd, Oxford.
- Chambers R, Schwartz A and Boath E (2002) *Beating Stress in the NHS*. Radcliffe Medical Press, Oxford.
- Lilley R (2002) *An A–Z of Management for Healthcare Professionals*. Radcliffe Medical Press, Oxford.
- Lilley R (2004) *The New GP Contract*. Radcliffe Publishing Ltd, Oxford.
- Lilley R and Lambden P (2005) *Making Sense of Risk Management: a workbook for primary care* (2e). Radcliffe Publishing Ltd, Oxford.
- Middleton J (2000) *The Team Guide to Communication*. Radcliffe Medical Press, Oxford.
- NHS Confederation (2005) *The NHS in England 2005/6: a pocket guide*. The NHS Confederation, London.
- Phillips A (2001) *Healthcare Management Dictionary*. Radcliffe Medical Press, Oxford.
- Phillips A (2001) *The Business Planning Tool Kit. A workbook for the primary care team*. Radcliffe Medical Press, Oxford.
- Phillips A (2002) *Assertiveness and the Manager's Job*. Radcliffe Medical Press, Oxford.
- Phillips A (2002) *Communication and the Manager's Job*. Radcliffe Medical Press, Oxford.
- Pietroni R (2001) *The Toolbox for Portfolio Development: a practical guide for the primary healthcare team*. Radcliffe Medical Press, Oxford.
- Talbot L and Pora D (2003) *Primary Care Training and Development: the toolkit*. Radcliffe Medical Press, Oxford.
- Tranberg H and Rashbass J (2004) *Medical Records: use and abuse*. Radcliffe Publishing Ltd, Oxford.

Hippocratic Oath

I swear by Apollo the physician, and Aesculapius and health and All-Heal and all the gods and goddesses, that, according to my ability and judgement, I shall keep this Oath and stipulation – to reckon him who taught me this Art equally dear to me as my parents, to share my substance with him and relieve his necessities if required, to look upon his offspring as my own brothers, and to teach them this Art, if they shall wish to learn it, without fee or stipulation, and that by precept, lecture and every other mode of instruction, I shall impart knowledge of the Art to my own sons, and those of my teachers, and to disciplines bound by stipulations and oath, according to the law of medicine but to none others. I will follow that system which, according to my judgement, I consider for the benefit of my patients and abstain from whatever is harmful for them. I shall give no deadly medicine to anyone if asked, nor suggest any such consent and in like manner I shall not advise a woman to procure abortion. With purity and holiness I shall pass my life and practise my Art. Into whatever houses I enter, I shall go into them for the benefit of the sick. Whatever I see or hear, in the life of men, which ought not to be spoken abroad, I shall not divulge, as reckoning that all such should be kept secret.

Training programmes

The following is a selection of the principal nationally validated training programmes of relevance to receptionists and secretaries working in the field of healthcare.

Radcliffe Publishing Ltd

18 Marcham Road
Abingdon
Oxon OX14 2AA
Tel: 01235 528820

Practice Receptionist Programmes for Administrative Staff in Primary Care
Managing the Practice
Dental Receptionist Programmes

Certificates are awarded on satisfactory completion of these training programmes, which are also available in a format for distance/open learning.

Association of Medical Secretaries, Practice Managers, Administrators and Receptionists (AMSPAR)

Tavistock House North
Tavistock Square
London WC1H 9LN
Tel: 0207 387 6005

AMSPAR Certificate in Medical Terminology
AMSPAR Certificate in General Practice Reception
AMSPAR Receptionist Programme
AMSPAR Certificate in Hospital Reception
AMSPAR Diploma in Medical Secretarial Studies
AMSPAR Intermediate Diploma in Medical Reception
AMSPAR Advanced Diploma in Medical Secretarial Studies
AMSPAR Diploma in Primary Care Management
AMSPAR Diploma in Primary Care Management (Open Learning) (from 2005)

OCR (Oxford, Cambridge and RSA) Examinations Board

Westwood House
Westwood Way
Coventry CV4 8HS
Tel: 01203 470033

Medical Shorthand Speed Test, 80, 90, 100 wpm
Medical Audio Transcription
Medical Audio Transcription (Parts 1 and 2, Modular Award)
Medical Word Processing (Parts 1 and 2, Modular Award)

Pitman Examinations Institute

Medical Shorthand, 80, 90, 100 wpm

NHS Institute for Learning, Skills and Innovation (NILSI)

The NHS University has merged with the Modernisation Agency to form NILSI. At the time of going to press the NHSU and the Department of Health have not specified which NHSU training projects will be continued. The Department of Health has stated that the new agency will improve on the work of the NHSU by providing the NHS with a single agency for service, technology and personnel development, particularly in providing broad training to junior and support staff.

Medical terminology

Some components of words referring to body structures

A knowledge of these words will help you to deduce the meanings of many of the medical terms you hear and see in the course of your work.

Component of word	Pertaining to
aden	gland
angi	vessels (especially blood vessels)
arthr	joint(s)
aur	ear(s)
cardi	heart
caud	tail
cephal	head
cheil	lip(s)
chole	biliary system
cholecyst	gall-bladder
chondr	cartilage
col	colon
cyst	bladder
derm	skin
enter	intestine
fibr	fibrous tissue
gastr	stomach
gloss	tongue
haem or hem	blood
hepat	liver
hyster	uterus
labi	lips
lymph	lymphatic system
mamm, mast	breast(s)
myel	bone marrow or spinal cord
myo	muscle(s)
nephr	kidney(s)
ocul, ophthal	eye
onych	nails
or	mouth
orch, orchid	testes

os, oste	bone(s)
ot	ear(s)
pneumon	lung(s)
proct	rectum
pyel	kidney pelvis
ren	kidneys
rhin	nose
salping	uterine tubes
sial	salivary glands
spondyl	vertebra(ae)

Suffixes

Suffix	Meaning	Example	Definition
-algia	pain	arthralgia	joint pain
-ac	pertaining to	cardiac	pertaining to the heart
-al		chondral	pertaining to cartilage
-ar		vascular	relating to blood vessels
-ary		coronary	pertaining to the heart
-ic	referring to	pelvic	relating to the pelvis
-ory		sensory	pertaining to feeling
-ous	denoting	cutaneous	pertaining to the skin
-aemia	blood	hyperglycaemia	high blood sugar
-cele	swelling, hernia	cystocele	hernia of the bladder
		myelocele	protrusion of spinal cord through vertebrae
-centesis	puncture	paracentesis	puncture of a cavity
		thoracocentesis	aspiration of pleural cavity
-cyte	cell	leucocyte	white blood cell
-desis	binding, fixation	arthodesis	surgical fixation of a joint
-dynia	pain	pleurodynia	pain in the intercostal muscles
-ectasis	dilation	atelectasis	abnormal dilation of bronchus or bronchi
-ectomy	removal, excision	tonsillectomy	removal of tonsils
-genic	origin	bronchogenic	originating in bronchi
-genesis	forming, producing	pathogenesis	producing disease
-gram	tracing, recording	venogram	recording (X-ray) of veins
-graphy	process of recording	arteriography	X-ray of arteries
-iasis	condition of, presence, formation of	lithiasis	formation of stones
		cholelithiasis	formation of stones in gall-bladder
-itis	inflammation	carditis	inflammation of heart

		rhinitis	inflammation of mucous membrane of nose
-logy	study of	cytology	study of cells
-malacia	softening	osteomalacia	softening of bone
-megaly	enlargement	cardiomegaly	enlargement of heart
-oid	like, resembling	osteoid	like bone
-oma	tumour	osteoma	tumour of bone
-osis	disease, abnormal condition	spondylosis	disease of spine
-pathy	disease	myelopathy	disease of spinal cord
-penia	lack of	leucopenia	deficiency of white blood cells
-phasia	ability to speak	dysphasia	difficulty in speaking
-phagia	ability to swallow	dysphagia	difficulty in swallowing
-phobia	fear of	agoraphobia	fear of open spaces
-pnoea	breath	dyspnoea	difficulty in breathing
-rrhage	a bursting out	haemorrhage	an escape of blood from the vessels
-stasis	arrest, or cessation, a halting	haemostasis	the arrest of a flow of blood
-trophy	nourishment	atrophy	to waste away
-uria	pertaining to urine	haematuria	presence of blood in urine

Prefixes

Prefix	Meaning	Example	Definition
a-	absence, lack of	amnesia	loss of memory
ab-	from, away from	abduct	move away from mid-line of body
ad-	to, towards	adduct	move towards the mid-line of body
an-	absence, lack of	anaesthesia	loss of sensation
ante-	before	antepartum	before delivery
anti-	against	antiseptic	agent used against bacteria
brady-	slow	bradycardia	slow heart beat
contra-	opposite	contralateral	opposite side
circum-	around	cirumoral	around the mouth
co-/com-/ con-	with/joined together/ beside	co-habit	dwelling together
		compound	to mix or fuse
		congenital	present at birth
di-	disengage	diarthrosis	to separate from a joint
dia-	through, by means of	diastasis	separation, especially of skull sutures
ec-	out from	ectopic	not in normal place
endo	within	endometrium	lining of the uterus
exo-	outside	exogenous	produced outside

hypo-	beneath	hypotension	below normal blood pressure
infra-	under	infrapatellar	under the kneecap
inter-	between	intercostal	between the ribs
intra-	within	intracellular	within a cell
mega-	large, abnormally enlarged	megacolon	abnormally large (dilated) colon
micro-	abnormally small	microscopic	visible only with aid of microscope
onc-	pertaining to tumours	oncology	scientific study of tumours
para-	near, beside	paravertebral	beside the vertebra
peri-	around	pericardium	around the heart
pre-	in front of/before	prenatal	before birth
pro-	in front of	prognosis	forecast (of course of disease)
retro-	backwards	retroflexion	bending backward
sym-	beside	symphysis	growing together
syn-	along	synapse	joining of two neurones
tachy-	rapid	tachycardia	rapid heart beat
trans-	across	transurethral	through the urethra

Some of the most commonly used abbreviations

AID	artificial insemination by donor
AIDS	acquired immune deficiency syndrome
APH	antepartum haemorrhage
ASD	atrial septal defect
ASD	autistic spectrum disorders
bd	twice per day
BI	bony injury
BP	blood pressure, *British Pharmacopoeia*
CDH	congenital dislocation of the hip
CSF	cerebrospinal fluid
CNS	central nervous system
CT	computed tomography
CAT	computed axial tomography
CSU	catheter specimen of urine
CVP	central venous pressure
CVS	cardiovascular system
D&C	dilatation and curettage (uterine)
DLE	disseminated lupus erythematosus
DNA	did not attend (or deoxyribonucleic acid)
DS	disseminated sclerosis
DU	duodenal ulcer
D&V	diarrhoea and vomiting
DVT	deep vein thrombosis
DXRT	deep X-ray therapy
ECG	electrocardiography

EDD	expected date of delivery
ENT	ear, nose and throat
ESR	erythrocyte sedimentation rate
EUA	examination under anaesthetic
FB	foreign body
FHH	fetal heart heard
FDIU	fetal death *in utero*
GU	gastric ulcer
Hb	haemoglobin
HRT	hormone replacement therapy
IM	intramuscular
Ig	immunoglobulin
ISQ	in status quo (unchanged)
IUCD	intrauterine contraceptive device
IUD	intrauterine death or intrauterine (contraceptive) device
IV	intravenous
LB	loose body
MI	myocardial infarct
MRI	magnetic resonance imaging
MS	multiple sclerosis or mitral stenosis
MSU	midstream specimen of urine
NAD	no abnormality detected
NAI	non-accidental injury
NG	new growth
NYD	not yet diagnosed
OA	osteoarthritis
OT	occupational therapy
PET	positron emission tomography
PID	prolapsed intervertebral disc
PM	post-mortem
POP	plaster of Paris
PPH	postpartum haemorrhage
PR	per (through) the rectum
PUO	pyrexia of unknown origin
PV	per (through) the vagina
RA	rheumatoid arthritis
RBC	red blood cell
RH	rhesus factor
SMR	submucous resection of nasal septum
SOB	shortness of breath
SOL	space-occupying lesion
SOS	if necessary
SPECT	single photon emission computed tomography
TB	tuberculosis or tubercle bacilli
tds	three times a day
THR	total hip replacement
TPR	temperature, pulse and respiration
Ts & As	tonsils and adenoids
TUR	transurethral resection (of prostate)
UTI	urinary tract infection
VD	venereal disease

VVs	varicose veins
WBC	white blood cells
WR	Wassermann reaction
XR	X-ray

Medical symbols

♀	male
♂	female
#	fracture
Δ	diagnosis
R$_x$	recipe (for prescription – 'take thou')
+ve	positive
–ve	negative
c̄	with
s̄	without
1/7	one day
3/7	three days
1/52	one week
1/12	one month

Abbreviations used in prescribing

Abbreviation	Latin equivalent	English meaning
aa	ana	of each the amount
ac	ante cibum	before food
bd (or bid)	bis die (bis in die)	twice daily
c̄	cum	with
hn	hac nocte	tonight
mane	mane	in the morning
mdu	more dicta utendus	as previously directed
m et n	mane et nocte	morning and night
nocte	nocte	at night
om	omni mane	every morning
on	omni nocte	every night
pc	post cibum	after food
prn	pro re nata	whenever necessary
qds	quater die sumendum	four times a day
qid	quater in die	four times a day
sos	si opus sit	if necessary
stat	statim	immediately
td (or tid)	ter die (ter in die)	three times a day
tds	ter die sumendum	three times a day

Investigations

Digestive system

Test	Reason for test
Oral cytology	Detection of early cancer in the elderly
Oesophagoscopy (visual inspection of oesophagus)	Investigation of tumours, strictures; removal of foreign bodies
Gastroscopy (visual inspection of stomach)	Investigation of abnormalities (e.g. gastric ulcer, carcinoma)
Liver function tests (LFTs)	Liver disease; obstructive jaundice; haemolytic jaundice
Endoscopic retrograde cholangio-pancreatography (ERCP)	Detection of pancreatic cancer
Glucose tolerance tests (GTTs)	To test the patient's ability to stabilise his or her blood level
Laparoscopy (visual inspection of abdominal cavity)	Investigation of lower abdominal pain
Proctoscopy (visual inspection of anal canal and lower rectum)	Detection of haemorrhoids or growths
Colonoscopy (visual inspection of colon)	Investigation of malignant changes or for biopsy
Sigmoidoscopy (visual inspection of sigmoid colon)	Detection of growths; ulcerative colitis
Examination of faeces	Diagnosis of gastric/duodenal ulcers/carcinoma

Investigations and tests relating to haematology and blood transfusion

Test	Reason for test
Haemoglobin (Hb) estimation	Detection of abnormalities (e.g. polycythaemia, anaemia)
Red blood cell count (RBC)	
Haematocrit or packed cell volume (PCV)	Routine blood investigations for presence of abnormalities
Mean corpuscular haemoglobin (MCH)	
Mean corpuscular haemoglobin concentration (MCHC)	
Erythrocyte sedimentation rate (ESR)	A test to screen for systematic disease, or progress of disease (e.g. inflammatory and autoimmune disease, malignancy, serious infection)

White blood cell count (WBC)	Detection of disease and infection (e.g. pneumonia, leukaemia, appendicitis)
Platelet count	Detection of disease, trauma, infection, inflammation, malignancy
Clotting time	To test extrinsic clotting system in diagnosis of haemophilia, obstructive jaundice, etc.
Prothrombin ratio	Investigation of haemorrhagic disorders, liver disease
Paul Bunnell	To diagnose infective mononucleosis (glandular fever)
Monospot	To diagnose infective mononucleosis (glandular fever)
Rose–Waaler (RA)	To diagnose rheumatoid arthritis
Latex fixation test	To diagnose rheumatoid arthritis
Antinuclear factor/antibody (ANF/ANA)	To diagnose systemic lupus erythematosus

Bacterial tests on blood

Widal reaction (WR)	Diagnosis of typhoid/paratyphoid and brucellosis
VDRL	Diagnosis of venereal disease
TPHA	Diagnosis of venereal disease
WR	Diagnosis of venereal disease
GCFT	Diagnosis of venereal disease
Guthrie's test	Estimation of blood level of phenylketonuria (PKU) in babies

Musculoskeletal system

Disorders of bones and joints give rise to pain, deformity, swelling of bone and tissues, limitation of movement and secondary muscle wasting.

X-ray investigation is of value in diagnosis and assessment of the response to treatment. Bone scanning is increasingly being used for detection of malignant conditions in bone.

Test	Reason for test
Arthroscopy (visual inspection of knee joint)	Diagnosis of disease/injury to interior of joint
Electromyography	Detection of muscular disorders (e.g. muscular dystrophy, myasthenia gravis and myotonia)
Myelography	Detection of spinal lesions (e.g. tumours and prolapsed intervertebral disc)
Radiculography	Similar procedure to myelography, used to investigate the lumbosacral nerve roots

(see also Miscellaneous investigations)

Cardiovascular system

Test	Reason for test
Blood pressure (BP)	To detect disease Hypertension – abnormally high blood pressure Hypotension – abnormally low blood pressure
Angio-cardiography (injection of dye through catheter enabling X-ray of heart structure)	Detection of abnormalities of the heart and blood vessels
Electrocardiography (ECG) (recording of electrical activity of the heart)	To investigate heart disorders (e.g. coronary thrombosis, heart block)
Echocardiography	Diagnosis of valvular disease and pericardial effusion

Respiratory system

Test	Reason for test
Rhinoscopy (examination of interior of nose)	Removal of tissue for histology, or swab taken for bacteriology
Laryngoscopy	Examination of vocal cords, larynx and epiglottis, for growths and infections
Bronchoscopy (visual inspection of bronchi)	Diagnosis of growths; tissue removal for biopsy
Sputum examination	Examination of sputum for blood, parasites, etc.
Pleural fluid	Detection of malignancy, chest injury, emphysema, heart failure

Lung function tests

Vital capacity of lungs (maximum amount of air which can be expired)	Measurement of amount of air expired by a patient – diminished in lung disease
Wright's peak-flow meter	Detection of lung disease

Nervous system

Test	Reason for test
Lumbar puncture	Examination of cerebrospinal fluid (CSF) and diagnosis of certain diseases of nervous system

Romberg's sign	Test for co-ordination, used in diagnosis of multiple sclerosis, cerebral tumour, etc.
Kernig's sign	Diagnosis of meningitis, cerebral haemorrhage or meningism
Electroencephalogram (EEG)	Investigation of epileptic conditions and location of cerebral lesions
Electromyogram (EMG) (recording of electrical activity in a muscle)	Investigation of disease
Knee jerk	Detection of disease of nervous system

Pupil reflexes

Reaction to light	Detection of diseases of central nervous system

Eye tests

Optic discs	Detection of disease of central nervous system
Snellen's test	Measurement of extent of field of vision
Refraction tests	To correct defective vision by prescription of correct lens

Hearing tests

Audiometric tests	Determination of degree and type of hearing
Weber's test (tuning fork)	To distinguish between middle-ear and nerve deafness
Rinne's test	Detection of middle-ear deafness
Auriscopy (visual examination of middle ear)	Detection of infection and disease

Urinary system

Test	Reason for test
Routine laboratory examination	Detection of urinary infections, pyelonephritis, haematuria (blood in urine)
Mid-stream urine specimen (MSU)	Nephritis, presence of parasites – tropical disease

Test for protein	Presence of protein in urine (albuminuria)
Test for sugar	Presence of sugar in urine (glycosuria)
Test for ketones	Presence of ketones in urine (ketonuria)
Test for blood	Presence of blood in urine (haematuria)

Renal efficiency tests

Blood urea	Impairment of renal function
Urea clearance test	To indicate extent of kidney damage
Cystoscopy (visual inspection of bladder)	Detection of disease of bladder; for biopsy of tissue/tumour
Intravenous pyelogram (IVP)	To test renal function; to demonstrate hydronephrosis, renal calculi, hydronephroma, etc.
Renal biopsy	Specimen sent for histology

Pregnancy tests

Oestriol examination	Assessment of both placental and fetal function
Toxaemia of pregnancy	Urine tested for protein – to confirm condition
Amniocentesis	Estimation of fetal maturity; detection of fetal defects, etc.
Cervical smear	Early diagnosis of cancer; detection of infection and other conditions
Vaginal swab	To detect cause of vaginal discharge

Endocrine glands

Test	Reason for test
Thyroid function tests (TFTs)	Assessment of functioning of thyroid glands
Protein-bound iodine (PBI)	Measurement of thyroid function

X-ray investigations

Test	Reason for test
Barium swallow	Detection of lesions of oesophagus; demonstration of hiatus hernia
Barium meal	Detection of lesions of stomach and duodenum
Barium meal with follow-through	Detection of lesions of small and large intestines
Barium enema	Detection of disease and obstruction of the bowel
Double-contrast radiography	Detection of small changes in gastric mucosa (e.g. early carcinoma)
Cholecystography	To demonstrate presence of gallstones
Intravenous cholangiogram	To demonstrate bile duct obstruction due to growth or stones
Arthrogram	To outline joint cavity
Bone scan	Detection of secondary tumours
Angiography	Demonstration of obstruction, aneurysm or abnormal course (of blood vessel)
Aortogram	Angiogram of aorta
Arteriogram	Angiogram of arteries
Venogram	Angiogram of veins
Bronchography	Diagnosis of bronchiectasis and other bronchial abnormalities
Lung scan	Demonstration of tumours
Mammography	Detection of early malignancy of breast
Myelogram	Examination of spinal cord for obstruction and other defects
Encephalogram	Detection of cerebral tumours
Ventriculogram	To confirm cerebral tumour

Skin tests

Mantoux test	Skin test for sensitivity to TB by dilute intradermal injection of tuberculin
Heaf test	Similar to Mantoux, but using multiple-puncture technique
Kveim test	Intradermal injection to diagnose sarcoidosis

Miscellaneous investigations

Radiography

X-rays are one of the most frequently requested investigations used by physicians. They are painless unless used in conjunction with a contrast medium, which may cause discomfort. They are also quick and easy to perform, but may be frightening for the patient.

X-rays are a form of electromagnetic energy of a short wavelength which have the ability to penetrate tissues.

Plain X-rays are commonly performed on the chest, the abdomen, the skull and limbs in order to study bones for bone disease, fractures, etc. Contrast media may be used to visualise soft tissues and organs.

Ultrasonography (ultrasound)

Ultrasound is a non-invasive diagnostic procedure used to view body structures. It is convenient, safe and a comparatively inexpensive investigation. It does not use ionising radiation and is therefore safer than radiography. Ultrasound examinations are performed on the following structures:

- the brain – electroencephalography

- the arteries and veins

- the heart – echocardiography

- the kidney, liver and pelvis.

In obstetrics, the main use of ultrasonography is to demonstrate fetal size and growth, and the position of the placenta.

Computed tomography

Computed tomography (CT) scanning is an X-ray technique which uses a computer to reconstruct an image of a layer of tissue in the body. The CT scanner can image the three main cavities of the body (head, thorax and abdomen). It is mainly used for detecting lesions such as tumours and cysts in the body.

A second-generation CT system has evolved which produces three-dimensional images of the body. These images allow doctors to examine, for example, a person's brain as if it were being held in their hands.

Nuclear magnetic resonance imaging (NMRI)

This form of investigation is now widely used in medicine, and is often referred to as MRI. It uses radio-frequency radiation in the presence of a magnetic field to produce anatomical sections of the human body.

It is a non-invasive technique, it does not use ionising radiation, and it penetrates the structures of the body. In contrast with CT scanning, MRI can provide images in any anatomical plane.

Radioisotope scanning

A radioactive isotope is an unstable isotope which decays or disintegrates, emitting radiation or energy as it does so. The energy source is inside the patient and is given either orally or intravenously.

Radioisotopic scans are performed in order to detect malfunction or abnormalities of bones, lungs, brain, heart, kidneys, gall-bladder, spleen and endocrine glands.

Thermography

This is a technique which measures and records heat energy from the skin surface. It is non-invasive and causes no discomfort. Films are taken in much the same way as a photograph. Plates containing the films are placed on the skin and changes of skin temperature are reflected on a colour map.

Thermography is mainly used to detect lesions of the breast, to evaluate drug therapy, and to diagnose spinal root compression, and it may be used to assess the progress of wound healing.

Tomography

This is a technique in which a single layer of tissue is examined. This is achieved by blurring the image of the tissues above and below the layer of tissue to be studied when the X-ray is taken.

Fluoroscopy

Fluoroscopy enables the function of organs to be directly visualised in motion on a fluorescent screen (e.g. the heart beat, movement of the diaphragm and motility of the gastrointestinal tract can be observed and recorded).

Immunisation schedules

Recommended immunisations for children

The new routine vaccination schedule includes the pneumococcal vaccine which will be added to the childhood immunisation programme during 2006.

When is the immunisation due?	Which immunisation?	Type
At two months	• Polio	By mouth
	• Hib • Diphtheria • Tetanus • Whooping cough (pertussis) • Pneumococcal vaccine	One injection
At three months	• Polio	By mouth
	• Hib • Diphtheria • Tetanus • Whooping cough	One injection
	• Meningitis C	One injection
At four months	• Polio	By mouth
	• Hib • Diphtheria • Tetanus • Whooping cough • Pneumococcal vaccine	One injection
At 12 months	• Hib • Meningitis C	One injection
At 13 months	• Measles • Mumps • Rubella	One injection
	• Pneumococcal vaccine	One injection

The Department of Health advises that children should not be given separate measles, mumps and rubella vaccines in place of MMR, since there is no evidence of benefit and a clear risk of harm from following such a practice.

Cont

3 to 5 years (usually before the child starts school)	• Measles • Mumps • Rubella	One injection
	• Diphtheria • Tetanus • Whooping cough (acellular pertussis) (DTaP)	One injection
	• Polio	By mouth
10 to 14 years (sometimes shortly after birth)	• Heaf test and BCG (tuberculosis)	Skin test followed by one injection
School leavers 13 to 18 years	• Tetanus	One injection
	• Polio	By mouth

© 2001 Crown Copyright

Recommended immunisations for adults

Disease	Frequency	Method
Tetanus toxoid (for immunised adults who have received five doses, booster doses are not recommended unless at the time of tetanus- prone injury)	Booster every 10 years	One injection, or three at monthly intervals for those previously unvaccinated
Polio	Booster every 10 years until age 40 years	By mouth (OPV)
For at-risk groups		
Influenza	Annually (especially for the elderly)	Injection
Hepatitis B	Booster every 3–5 years	Injections (in first instance, three over 6 months, followed by blood test)

Vaccinations for foreign travel

Travellers to hot climates and developing countries should be given immunisations and anti-malarial advice according to up-to-date recommendations, which can be found in the *Pulse* and *MIMS* charts which are published monthly, and the patient's previous immunisation status.

Incubation periods of some infectious diseases

The incubation period is the interval between the time of primary infection or contact with an infected person and the appearance of the disease. The following information is only a guide, as in some instances some of the diseases have been found to have an incubation period outside the stated range.

Disease or causative organism	Incubation period
Amoebic dysentery	1–4 weeks
Bacillus cereus enteritis	1–5 hours
Botulism	2 hours – 8 days (usually 12–36 hours)
Brucellosis	1–8 weeks (usually 2–3 weeks)
Campylobacter enteritis	1–11 days (usually 2–5 days)
Chicken-pox	10–21 days (usually 14–15 days)
Cholera	2–48 hours
Dysentery	1–7 days (usually 1–3 days)
German measles (rubella)	14–21 days
Infective jaundice (hepatitis A)	14–42 days
Hepatitis B	42 days – 6 months
Lassa fever	3–17 days
Legionnaire's disease	2–10 days
Leptospirosis	4–19 days (usually 7–12 days)
Malaria	8–25 days
Measles	7–21 days (usually 10–14 days)
Mumps	12–28 days (usually 16–18 days)
Polio	10–15 days
Rabies	2 weeks–5 years (usually 20–90 days)
Salmonella enteritis	6–72 hours
Scarlet fever	2–5 days
Typhoid fever	7–21 days
Whooping cough	5–21 days
Yellow fever	3–6 days

Abbreviations of qualifying degrees and further qualifications

ABPN	Association of British Psychiatric Nurses
AIHA	Association of the Institute of Hospital Administration
AIMLS	Association of the Institute of Medical Laboratory Sciences
BAc	Bachelor of Acupuncture
BAO	Bachelor of the Art of Obstetrics
BC, BCh, BChir	Bachelor of Surgery
BM	Bachelor of Medicine
BS, ChB, CChir	Bachelor of Surgery
BSc	Bachelor of Science
BSc (Soc Sci Nurs)	Bachelor of Nursing
CCFP	Certificate of the College of Family Practitioners
ChD	Doctor of Surgery
CM, ChM	Master of Surgery
CPH	Certificate in Public Health
CTCM&H	Certificate in Tropical Community Medicine and Hygiene
DA	Diploma in Anaesthetics
DAvMed	Diploma in Aviation Medicine
DCCH	Diploma in Child and Community Health
DCH	Diploma in Child Health
DCh	Doctor of Surgery
DCP	Diploma in Clinical Pathology
DCPath	Diploma of the College of Pathologists
DCR	Diploma of the College of Radiologists
DDR	Diploma in Diagnostic Radiology
DDS	Doctor of Dental Surgery
DFHom	Diploma of the Faculty of Homeopathy
DFM	Diploma in Forensic Medicine
DGM	Diploma in Geriatric Medicine
DHyg	Doctor of Hygiene
DIH	Diploma in Industrial Health
Dip GU Med	Diploma in Genitourinary Medicine
DLO	Diploma in Laryngology and Otology
Dip Med Rehab	Diploma in Medical Rehabilitation
DM	Doctor of Medicine

DMR	Diploma in Medical Radiology
DMRT	Diploma in Medical Radiotherapy
DN	Diploma in Nursing, District Nurse
DO	Diploma in Ophthalmology
DObstRCOG	Diploma in Obsterics of the Royal College of Obstetricians and Gynaecologists
DOMS	Diploma in Ophthalmological Medicine and Surgery
DPH	Diploma in Public Health
DPM	Diploma in Psychological Medicine
DR	Diploma in Radiology
DrAc	Doctor of Acupuncture
DS	Doctor of Surgery
DSc	Doctor of Science
DTM&H	Diploma in Tropical Medicine and Hygiene
En(G)	Enrolled Nurse (General)
En(M)	Enrolled Nurse (Mental)
FCGP	Fellow of the College of General Practitioners
FCOphth	Fellow of the College of Ophthalmology
FCPath	Fellow of the College of Pathologists
FDS	Fellow of Dental Surgery
FFA	Fellow of the Faculty of Anaesthetists
FFARCS	Fellow of the Faculty of Anaesthetists of the Royal College of Surgeons
FFHom	Fellow of the Faculty of Homeopathy
FFR	Fellow of the Faculty of Radiologists
FIBiol	Fellow of the Institute of Biology
FICS	Fellow of the International College of Surgeons
FLCO	Fellow of the London College of Osteopathy
FPS	Fellow of the Pharmaceutical Society
FRC Anaesth	Fellow of the Royal College of Anaesthetists
FRCGP	Fellow of the Royal College of General Practitioners
FRCN	Fellow of the Royal College of Nursing
FRCOG	Fellow of the Royal College of Obstetricians and Gynaecologists
FRCP	Fellow of the Royal College of Physicians of London
FRCPE	Fellow of the Royal College of Physicians of Edinburgh (may also be written as FRCPEd, FRCPEdin)
FRCPS	Fellow of the Royal College of Physicians and Surgeons
FRCPath	Fellow of the Royal College of Pathologists
FRCPsych	Fellow of the Royal College of Psychiatrists
FRCR	Fellow of the Royal College of Radiologists
FRCS	Fellow of the Royal College of Surgeons of England
FRCSE	Fellow of the Royal College of Surgeons of Edinburgh
FRIPHH	Fellow of the Royal Institute of Public Health and Hygiene
FRS	Fellow of the Royal Society
FRSH	Fellow of the Royal Society of Health
HVCert	Health Visitors Certificate
LAH	Licentiate of Apothecaries Hall, Dublin
LDS	Licentiate in Dental Surgery
LM	Licentiate in Midwifery
LRCP	Licentiate of the Royal College of Physicians

LSA	Licentiate of the Society of Apothecaries
MAO	Master of the Art of Obstetrics
MB	Bachelor of Medicine
MB ChB	Bachelor of Medicine Bachelor of Surgery
MC, MCh, MChir	Master of Surgery
MChD	Master of Dental Surgery
MChOrth	Master of Orthopaedic Surgery
MClinPsychol	Master of Clinical Psychology
MCommH	Master of Community Health
MCPath	Member of College of Pathology
MCPS	Member of College of Physicians and Surgeons
MD	Doctor of Medicine
MDS	Master of Dental Surgery
MFCP	Member of the Faculty of Community Physicians
MFHom	Member of the Faculty of Homeopathy
MHyg	Master of Hygiene
MIH	Master of Industrial Health
MLCOM	Member of the London College of Osteopathic Medicine
MMed	Master of Medicine
MMSA	Master of Midwifery of Society of Apothecaries
MO&G	Master of Obstetrics and Gynaecology
MOH	Medical Officer of Health
MPH	Master of Public Health
MPS	Member of the Pharmaceutical Society
MPsy	Master of Psychiatry
MPsychMed	Master of Psychological Medicine
MRad(D)	Master of Radiodiagnosis
MRad(T)	Master of Radiotherapy
MRCGP	Member of the Royal College of General Practitioners
MRCOG	Member of the Royal College of Obstetricians and Gynaecologists
MRCP	Member of the Royal College of Physicians
MRCPath	Member of the Royal College of Pathologists
MRCPsych	Member of the Royal College of Psychiatrists
MRCS	Member of the Royal College of Surgeons of England
MS	Master of Surgery
MSR(R)	Member of the Society of Radiography (Radiography)
MSR(T)	Member of the Society of Radiography (Radiotherapy)
RCM	Royal College of Midwives
RCN	Royal College of Nursing
RGN	Registered General Nurse
SEN	State Enrolled Nurse
SRN	State Registered Nurse
SRP	State Registered Physiotherapist

Other medical abbreviations (including job titles, organisations and non-clinical terms)

AHHRM	Association of Healthcare and Human Resource Management
AMSPAR	Association of Medical Secretaries, Practice Managers, Administrators and Receptionists
BACUP	British Association of Cancer-United Patients and their families and friends
BMA	British Medical Association
BMJ	*British Medical Journal*
BNF	*British National Formulary*
BP	*British Pharmacopoeia*
BPC	British Pharmaceutical Codex
BRCS	British Red Cross Society
CDO	Chief Dental Officer
CDSR	Cochrane Database of Systematic Reviews
CEM	cost-effectiveness-based medical decision making
CHD	coronary heart disease
CMHT	community mental health team
CME	continuing medical education
CMO	Chief Medical Officer
CNO	Chief Nursing Officer
CPA	Care Programme Approach
CPR	Child Protection Register
CSM	Committee on the Safety of Medicines
DDA	Dangerous Drugs Act
DH	Department of Health
DN	District Nurse
DSS	Department of Social Security
DSU	day surgery unit
EBM	evidence-based medicine
EBS	emergency bed service
ECHR	European Convention on Human Rights
ECR	extra-contractual referral
EDI	electronic data interchange
EPR	electronic paper record
FPA	Family Planning Association
GDP	General Dental Practitioner
GMC	General Medical Council
GMP	General Medical Practitioner
GMS	General Medical Services
HAZ	Health Action Zone
HCHS	hospital and community health services
HIMP	Health Improvement Programme
HTA	Health Technology Assessment
HV	Health Visitor
ICAS	Independent Complaints Advocacy Service

ICD	International Classification of Diseases
ICP	integrated care pathway
ICU	intensive care unit
IHSM	Institute of Health Services Management
ILA	Independent Learning Account
IMA	Independent Medical Adviser
IM&T	information management and technology
IPR	individual performance review
LMC	Local Medical Committee
MAAG	Medical Audit Advisory Group
MDU	Medical Defence Union
MHAC	Mental Health Act Commission
MHRT	Mental Health Review Tribunal
MIMS	*Monthly Index of Medical Specialities*
MPS	Medical Protection Society
MRC	Medical Research Council
MRI	magnetic resonance imaging
MSW	Medical Social Worker
NAO	National Audit Office
NBA	National Blood Authority
NBTS	National Blood Transfusion Service
NCAA	National Clinical Assessment Authority
NeLH	National electronic Library for Health
NHS	National Health Service
NHSLA	NHS Litigation Authority
NICE	National Institute for Clinical Excellence
NILSI	NHS Institute for Learning, Skills and Innovation
NMC	Nursing and Midwifery Council
NPSA	National Patient Safety Agency
NSF	National Service Framework
NTA	National Treatment Agency (Substance Misuse)
OCDMA	Oncology Data Managers Association
OHE	Office of Health Economics
OT	Occupational Therapist
OTC	over the counter
PACT	Prescribing Analyses and Costs
PALS	Patient Advocacy and Liaison Service
PCT	Primary Care Trust
PFI	Private Finance Initiative
PGEA	Postgraduate Educational Allowance
PHeL	Public Health electronic Library
PMS	Personal Medical Services
PPF	Patient and Public Involvement Forum
PPP	public–private partnership
PRINCE	PRojects IN Controlled Environment
PSA	public service agreement
QA	quality assurance
QALY	quality-adjusted life year
QCA	Qualifications Curriculum Authority
RCGP	Royal College of General Practitioners
RCN	Royal College of Nursing

RHA	regional health authority
RTA	road traffic accident
SHA	strategic health authority; special health authority
SHO	Senior House Officer
SI	Systeme International (units)
SLA	service level agreement
SMR	standardised mortality ratio
SNOMED	systemised nomenclature for medicine
SSI	Social Services Inspectorate
ST	Speech Therapist
TQM	Total Quality Management
WHO	World Health Organization

Useful addresses

Association of Medical Secretaries, Practice Administrators and Receptionists (AMSPAR)
Tavistock House North
Tavistock Square
London WC1H 9LN
Tel: 0207 387 6005

British Medical Association (BMA)
BMA House, Tavistock Square
London WC1H 9JP
Tel: 0207 387 4499

Council for Nursing and Midwifery (formerly UKCC)
23 Portland Place
London W1N 4JT
Tel: 020 7637 7181

Department of Social Security (DSS)
Eileen House, Elephant and Castle
London SE1 6BY
Tel: 0207 703 6380

Faculty of Public Health Medicine
4 St Andrew's Place
Regent's Park
London NW1 4LB
Tel: 0207 935 0243

General Medical Council (GMC)
Regents Place
360 Euston Road
London NW1 3JN
Tel: 0845 357 8001

GP Computer Centre
75 York Road
London SE1 7NT
Tel: 0207 620 0901

Health and Safety Executive and Health and Safety Commission
Rose Court
2 Southwark Bridge Road
London SE1 9HS
Tel: 020 7717 6000

Health Development Agency
10 Trevelyan House
30 Great Peter Street
London SW1P 2HW
Tel: 020 7227 5300

Health Service Ombudsman (Commissioner) for England
Millbank Tower
Millbank
London SW1 4QP
Tel: 0845 015 4033

Health Services Commissioner for Scotland
2nd Floor
11 Melville Crescent
Edinburgh EH3 7LU
Tel: 0131 225 7465

Health Services Commissioner for Wales
4th Floor, Pearl Assurance House
Greyfriars Road
Cardiff CF1 3AG
Tel: 01222 394621

Healthcare Commission
Finsbury Tower
103–5 Bunhill Row
London EC1X 8TG

Hospital Consultants and Specialists Association
The Old Court House
London Road
Ascot
Berkshire SL5 7EN
Tel: 01344 25052

Institute of Health and Care Development
St Bartholomew's Court
18 Christmas Street
Bristol BS1 5BT
Tel: 0207 929 1029

Institute of Health Services Management (IHSM)
7–10 Chandos Street
London W1M 9DE
Tel: 0207 460 7654

King's Fund
11–13 Cavendish Square
London W1G 0AN
Tel: 0207 307 2400

Medical Defence Union
3 Devonshire Place
London W1N 2EA
Tel: 0207 202 1500

Medical Protection Society
50 Hallam Street
London W1N 6DE
Tel: 0207 637 0541

Medical Research Council
220 Park Crescent
London W1N 4AL

Mental Health Act Commission
Maid Marian House
56 Houndsgate
Nottingham NG1 6BG
Tel: 0115 943 7100

Mental Welfare Commission for Scotland
Argyle House
3 Lady Lawson Street
Edinburgh EH3 9SH
Tel: 0131 226 6111

National Audit Office
159–197 Buckingham Palace Road
London SW1W 9SP
Tel: 020 7798 7000

National Council for Vocational Qualifications
222 Euston Road
London NW1 2BZ
Tel: 0207 387 3611

Royal College of General Practitioners
14 Princes Gate
London SW7 1PU
Tel: 0207 581 3232

Royal College of Nursing
20 Cavendish Square
London W1G 0RN
Tel: 0207 409 3333

Royal College of Obstetricians and Gynaecologists
27 Sussex Place
Regents Park
London NW1 4RG
Tel: 0207 262 5425

Royal College of Paediatrics and Child Health
50 Hallam Street
London W1N 6DE
Tel: 0207 307 5600

Royal College of Pathologists
2 Carlton House Terrace
London SW1Y 5AF
Tel: 0207 930 5861

Royal College of Physicians
11 St Andrew's Place
London NW1 4LE
Tel: 0207 935 1174

Royal College of Physicians of Edinburgh
9 Queen Street
Edinburgh EH2 1JQ
Tel: 0131 225 7324

Royal College of Physicians and Surgeons of Glasgow
232–242 St Vincent Street
Glasgow G2 5RJ
Tel: 0141 221 6072

Royal College of Psychiatrists
17 Belgrave Square
London SW1X 8PG
Tel: 0207 235 2351

Royal College of Surgeons of Edinburgh
Nicolson Street
Edinburgh EH8 9DW
Tel: 0131 556 6206

Royal College of Surgeons of England
35–43 Lincoln's Inn Fields
London WC2A 3PN
Tel: 0207 405 3474

Royal Pharmaceutical Society of Great Britain
1 Lambeth High Street
London SE1 7JN
Tel: 020 7735 9141

Royal Society of Medicine
1 Wimpole Street
London W1M 8AE
Tel: 0207 408 2119

RSA Examinations Board
Westwood Way
Coventry CV4 8HS
Tel: 01203 470033

The Royal Colleges and Faculties also have an 'umbrella' organisation which co-ordinates the work of the medical royal colleges:

The Academy of Medical Colleges
1 Wimpole Street
London W1M 8AE
Tel: 020 7290 3913

Statutory organisations

(including addresses and main functions)

This includes a selection of statutory bodies (government funded) which will be of interest and use to receptionists and secretaries working in healthcare, as their activities are related to health matters in the UK.

Audit Commission
1 Vincent Square, London SW1P 2PN. Tel: 0207 828 1212.
The Audit Commission promotes studies to ascertain efficiency, effectiveness and economy in local government and the NHS, and appoints auditors to the latter.

Clinical Standards Advisory Group
Room 19, Wellington House, 133–155 Waterloo Road, London SE1 8UG.
Tel: 0207 972 4918.
The Clinical Standards Advisory Group advises the NHS and its ministers on standards of clinical care of patients, and access to and availability of services.

Common Services Agency for the Scottish Health Service
Trinity Park House, South Trinity Road, Edinburgh EH5 3SE. Tel: 0131 552 6255.
This organisation provides the NHS in Scotland with a range of services.

Health and Safety Commission and Health and Safety Executive
2 Southwark Bridge Road, London SE1 9HS. Tel: 0207 717 6000.

The above organisations are both responsible for securing the health, safety and welfare of people and protecting the public against risks to health or safety from work activities.

Health Service Commissioner (Ombudsman)
11th Floor, Millbank Tower, Millbank, London SE1P 4QP. Tel: 0207 276 2035.
The Ombudsman investigates complaints about services provided by the NHS, and regularly reports to Parliament.

Medical Research Council (MRC)
20 Park Crescent, London W1N 4AL. Tel: 0207 636 5542.
The MRC promotes medical and related biological research to objectively improve healthcare. It also provides grants to individual scientists.

Medicines Control Agency (MCA)
Market Towcesters, Nine Elms Lane, London SE8 5NQ. Tel: 0207 273 0393.
The MCA is an executive agency of the Department of Health and ensures that branded and non-branded medicines in the UK meet the required quality and safety standards, thus safeguarding public health. It also applies the standards set out in the Medicines Act and the legislative criteria of the European Community.

Mental Health Act Commission
Maid Marian House, Houndsgate, Nottingham NG1 6BG. Tel: 0115 943 7000.
The Mental Health Act Commission is responsible for protecting the interests of patients who are detained under the Mental Health Act in England and Wales. Scotland and Ireland have their own separate regulations.

Mental Welfare Commission for Scotland
Argyle House, 3 Lady Lawson Street, Edinburgh EH3 9SH. Tel: 0131 222 6111.
The Commission has the same responsibilities for Scotland as the Mental Health Act Commission does for England and Wales.

National Audit Office (NAO)
157–197 Buckingham Palace Road, Victoria, London SW1W 9SP.
Tel: 0207 798 7000.
The NAO is accountable to Parliament. It audits all public expenditure (NHS and government expediture), and reports that money has been spent for the purpose intended and is accounted for.

National Blood Authority (NBA)
Oak House, Reeds Crescent, Watford WD1 1QH. Tel: 01923 486800.
The NBA was created in 1993 to manage all NHS blood services. It manages all regional transfusion services, ensures that blood and blood product supplies meet defined criteria, and that a high-quality, cost-effective supply of both blood and blood products is available to meet national requirements (this requires approximately two million donors).

Northern Ireland Central Services Agency for Health and Social Services
25–27 Adelaide Street, Belfast BT2 8FH. Tel: 01232 334431.
This agency provides a range of services to the Health and Social Services Boards and to family doctors.

Prescription Pricing Authority
Bridge House, 152 Pilgrim Street, Newcastle upon Tyne NE1 2SN.
Tel: 0191 232 5371.
The Prescription Pricing Authority calculates and makes payments to dispensing doctors and pharmacists in England for NHS prescriptions dispensed. They also provide information on dispensing and prescribing to health service authorities.

Public Health Laboratory Services (PHLS)
61 Colindale Avenue, London NW9 5DF. Tel: 0208 200 1295. (Headquarters Office)
The PHLS provides facilities for the prevention and diagnosis of communicable and infectious diseases. The headquarters in Colindale provide the site of the Laboratory and Communicable Diseases Surveillance Centre and the Central Public Health Laboratory. There are approximately 50 laboratories in England and Wales, which are led by the Colindale-based laboratory.

Standing Medical Advisory Committee and Standing Nursing and Midwifery Advisory Committee
Department of Health, Room 919, Wellington House, 135–155 Waterloo Road, London SE1 8UG. Tel: 0207 972 4919.

Standing Pharmaceutical Advisory Committee
Department of Health, Room 301, Richmond House, 79 Whitehall,
London SW1A 2NS. Tel: 0207 210 6117.
These three committees advise health ministers in England and Wales on matters relating to the medical, nursing, midwifery and pharmaceutical services.

Standing Committee on Postgraduate Medical and Dental Education (SCOPME)
1 Park Square, West London NW1 41J. Tel: 0207 935 3916.
SCOPME gives advice to the Secretary of State on continuing and postgraduate medical and dental education. There are separate councils for Scotland, Northern Ireland and Wales.

United Kingdom Transplant Support Service Authority
Fox Den Road, Stoke Gifford, Bristol BS12 6RR. Tel: 0117 975 7575.
This special health authority provides support services for the matching, allocation and distribution of donor organs for transplant.

Information and support groups

Addresses for other information and support groups can be found in the *Voluntary Agencies Directory* published by NCVO Publications, National Council for Voluntary Organisations, Regent's Wharf, 8 All Saints Street, London N1 9RL. Tel: 0207 713 6161. Telephone helpline numbers can be found in the *Telephone Helpline Directory* published by the Telephone Helplines Association, 4 Dean's Court, St Paul's Churchyard, London EC4V 5AA. Tel: 0207 248 3388.

Accident prevention in the home

Child Helpline Trust, Clarkes Court, 18–20 Farringdon Lane, London EC1R 3HA. Tel: 0207 608 3828.

Royal Society for the Prevention of Accidents, Edgbaston Park, 353 Bristol Road, Birmingham B5 7ST. Tel: 0121 248 2000.

Ageing

Age Concern England, Astral House, 268 London Road, Norbury, London SW16 4ER. Tel: 0208 765 7200.

AIDS

Communicable Diseases Surveillance Centre (PHLS), 61 Colindale Avenue, London NW9 5BQ. Tel: 0208 200 6868.

London Lighthouse, 111–117 Lancaster Road, London W11 1QT. Tel: 0207 792 1200.

Terence Higgins Trust Lighthouse (THTL), 52–54 Gray's Inn Road, London WC1X 8JU. Tel: 020 7831 0336.

Alcohol-related problems

Alcohol Accept (Alcohol and Substance Misuse), 724 Fulham Road, London SW6 5SE. Tel: 020 7371 7555.

Alcoholics Anonymous, PO Box 1, Stonebow House, Stonebow, York YO1 2NJ. Tel: 01904 644026.

Alcohol Concern, Waterbridge House, 32–36 Loman Street, London SE1 OEE. Tel: 0207 928 7377.

Alcohol Focus Scotland, 166 Buchanan Street, Glasgow G1 2NH. Tel: 0141 333 9677.

Alzheimer's disease

Alzheimer's Disease Society, Second Floor, Gordon House, 10 Greencoat Place, London SW1P 1PH. Tel: 0207 308 0808.

Ankylosing spondylitis

National Association for Ankylosing Spondylitis, PO Box 179, Mayfield, East Sussex TN20 6ZL. Tel: 01435 873527.

Arthritis

Arthritis Care, 18 Stephenson Way, London NW1 2HD. Tel: 0207 916 1500. Helpline: 0800 289170.

ASH (Action on Smoking and Health)

ASH, 109 Gloucester Place, London W1H 4EJ. Tel: 0207 035 3519.

Asthma

National Asthma Campaign, Providence House, Providence Place, London N1 ONT. Tel: 0207 226 2260.

Autism

National Autistic Society, 276 Willesden Lane, London NW2 5RB. Tel: 0208 451 1114.

Back pain

Back Care, 16 Elmtree Road, Teddington TW11 8TD. Tel: 0208 977 5474.

Blindness

Royal National Institute for the Blind, 105 Judd Street, London WC1H 9NE. Tel: 0207 388 2034.

Blood transfusion

National Blood Authority, Oak House, Reeds Crescent, Watford WD24 4QN. Tel: 08457 711 711.

Brain injuries

Headway, National Head Injuries Association, 4 King Edward Street, Nottingham NG1 1EW. Tel: 0115 924 0800.

Breast cancer care

Breast Cancer Care, Kiln House, 210 New King's Road, London SW6 4NZ. Tel: 0500 245345.

Brittle bone disease

Brittle Bone Society, 30 Guthrie Street, Dundee DD1 5BS. Tel: 01382 204446.

Cancer

Marie Curie Cancer Care, 89 Albert Embankment, London SE1 7TP. Tel: 0207 599 7777.

Macmillan Cancer Relief, 89 Albert Embankment, London SE1 7TP Tel: 0207 840 7840.

BACUP, 3 Bath Place, Rivington Street, London EC2A 3JR. Tel: 0207 696 9003.

Carers

Carers National Association, 25 Glasshouse Yard, London EC1A 4JS. Tel: 0207 490 8818.

Women's Royal Voluntary Service, Garden House, Milton Hill, Steventon, Oxon OX13 6AD. Tel: 01235 442900.

Care services

Counsel and Care, Twyman House, 16 Bonny Street, London NW1 9PG. Tel: 0207 267 6877.

Cerebral palsy

SCOPE, PO Box 833, Milton Keynes, MK12 5NY. Tel: 0207 619 7100.

Capability Scotland, 2 Corstorphine Road, Edinburgh EH12 6HP. Tel: 0131 337 9876.

Child adoption

British Agencies for Adoption and Fostering (BAAF), Skyline House, 200 Union Street, London SE1. Tel: 0207 593 2000.

Childbirth

National Childbirth Trust, Alexandra House, Oldham Terrace, Acton, London W3 6NH. Tel: 0208 992 6637.

Children

Action for Sick Children (National Association for the Welfare of Children in Hospital), Argyle House, 29–31 Euston Road, London NW1 2SD. Tel: 0207 833 2041.

National Society for the Prevention of Cruelty to Children (NSPCC), NSPCC National Centre, 42 Curtain Road, London EC2A 3NH. Tel: 0207 825 2500.

Coeliac disease

Coeliac Society of the United Kingdom, PO Box 220, High Wycombe, Buckinghamshire HP11 2HY. Tel: 01494 437278.

Colitis and Crohn's disease

National Association for Colitis and Crohn's Disease, PO Box 205, St Albans, Hertfordshire. Tel: 01727 844296.

Colostomy

British Colostomy Association, 15 Station Road, Reading, Berkshire RG1 1LG. Tel: 0118 939 1537.

Coronary heart disease

Coronary Prevention Group, 2 Taunton Street, London WC1H 0BT. Tel: 0207 927 2125.

Cystic fibrosis

Cystic Fibrosis Trust, 11 London Road, Bromley, Kent BR1 1BY. Tel: 0208 464 7211.

Deafness

Royal National Institute for Deaf People, 19–23 Featherstone Street, London EC1Y 8SL. Tel: 0207 296 8000.

Sense (National Deaf, Blind and Rubella Association), 11–13 Clifton Terrace, Finsbury Park, London N4 3RS. Tel: 0207 272 7774.

Sense Scotland, 43 Middlesex Street, Kinning Park, Glasgow G41 1EE. Tel: 0141 429 0294

National Deaf Children's Society, 15 Dufferin Street, London EC1Y 8UR. Tel: 0207 250 0123.

Dermatitis

National Eczema Society, Hill House, Highgate Hill, London N19 5ND.
Tel: 0207 281 3553.

Diabetes

Diabetes UK, 10 Park Way, London NW1 7AA.
Tel: 0207 424 1000.

Disabled living

Disabled Living Foundation, 380–384 Harrow Road, London W9 2HU.
Tel: 0207 289 6111.

British Red Cross UK, 44 Moorfields, London EC2Y 9AL.
Tel: 0870 170 7000.

Disability Scotland, Information Department, Princes House,
5 Shandwick Place, Edinburgh EH2 4RG. Tel: 0131 229 8632.

Motability, City Gate House, 22 Southwark Bridge Road, London SE1 9HB.
Tel: 0845 130 9177.

Royal Society for Disability and Rehabilitation (RADARO), 12 City Forum,
250 City Road, London EC1V 8AF. Tel: 0207 250 3222.

Shaftesbury Society, 16 Kingston Road, London SW19 1JZ. Tel: 0208 542 5550.

Donors

National Blood Transfusion Service. Tel: 0345 71171.

National Blood Authority, Oak House, Reeds Crescent, Watford,
Hertfordshire WD1 1QH. Tel: 01923 486800. The NBA manages all NHS blood
services, including the management of the 15 regional transfusion services.

HM Inspector of Anatomy, Department of Health, Wellington House,
133–155 Waterloo Road, London SE1 8UG. Tel: 0207 972 4918.

NHS Organ Donor Register, FREEPOST SWB 1474, Patchway, Bristol
BS34 8ZZ. Tel: 0845 6060 400.

Down's syndrome

Down's Syndrome Association, Langdon Down Centre, 2A Langdon Park,
Teddington TW11 9PS. Tel: 0845 230 0372.

Drug dependence

National helpline. Tel: 0800 776600.

Dyslexia

British Dyslexia Association, 98 London Road, Reading, Berkshire RG1 5AU.
Tel: 01734 668271.

Dysphasia

Speakability, 1 Royal Street, London SE1 7LL.
Tel: 0207 261 9572

Stroke Association, 240 City Road, London EC1V 2PR.
Tel: 0207 928 9542.

Dystonia

Dystonia Society, 46–47 Britton Street, London EC1M 5NA. Tel: 0207 489 5671.

Eating disorders

Eating Disorders Association, First Floor, Wensum House,
103 Prince of Wales Road, Norwich NR1 1DW. Tel: 01603 619090.
Helpline: 01603 621414.

Eclampsia and pre-eclampsia

Action on Pre-eclampsia (APEC), 84–88 Pinner Road, Harrow HA1 4HZ.
Tel: 0208 427 4217.

Eczema

see Dermatitis

Epilepsy

British Epilepsy Association, New Anstey House, Gateway Drive, Yeadon, Leeds
LS19 7XY. Tel: 0113 391 0300.

Epilepsy Association of Scotland, 48 Govan Road, Glasgow G51 1JL.
Tel: 0141 427 4911.

Family planning

Family Planning Association, 2–12 Pentonville Road, London N1 9FP.
Tel: 0207 837 5432.

First aid

British Red Cross, 44 Moorfields, London EC2Y 9AL.
Tel: 0870 170 7000.

St John's Ambulance, 27 St John's Lane, Clerkenwell, London EC1M 4DA.
Tel: 0870 170 7000.

St Andrew's Ambulance Association, Strachan House, 16 Torphichen Street,
Edinburgh EH3 8JB. Tel: 0131 229 5419.

Haemophilia

Haemophilia Society, 1st Floor, Petersham House, 57a Hatton Garden, London
EC1N 8JP. Tel: 0207 405 4824.

Huntington's chorea

Huntington's Disease Association, 108 Battersea High Street,
London SW18 3HP. Tel: 0207 223 7000.

Ileostomy

Ileostomy and Internal Bag Support Group, Peverill House, 1–5 Mill Road,
Ballycare, Co Antrim BT39 9DR. Tel: 0800 0184 724.

Laryngectomy

National Association of Laryngectomy Clubs (NALC), Ground Floor,
6 Rickett Street, Fulham, London SW6 1RU. Tel: 0207 381 9993.

Learning disability

Mental Health Foundation, 20 Upper Ground, London SE1 9QB.
Tel: 0207 535 7400.

British Institute of Learning Disabilities, Green Street, Kidderminster,
Worcestershire DY10 1JL. Tel: 01562 723010.

MENCAP (Royal Society for Mentally Handicapped Children and Adults),
123 Golden Lane, London EC1Y 0RT. Tel: 0207 454 0454.

ENABLE (Scottish Society for the Mentally Handicapped), 7 Buchanan Street,
Glasgow G1 3HL. Tel: 0141 226 4541.

Lupus

Lupus UK, St James House, Eastern Road, Romford, Essex RM1 3NH.
Tel: 01708 731251.

Medical accidents

Action for the Victims of Medical Accidents, 44 High Street, Croydon, Sussex
CR0 1YB. Tel: 0845 123 2352.

Meningitis

National Meningitis Trust, Fern House, Bath Road, Stroud GL5 3TJ.
Tel: 01453 7751738.

Mental health

MIND (National Association for Mental Health), Granta House,
15–18 Broadway, Stratford, London E15 4BQ. Tel: 0208 519 2122.

Mental Health Act Commission, Maid Marian House, 56 Houndsgate,
Nottingham NG1 6BG. Tel: 0115 943 100.

Migraine

Migraine Action Association (British Migraine Association), Unit 6,
Hay Lodge Business Park, Great Folds Road, Great Oakley, Northamptonshire
NN18 9AS. Tel: 01536 461333.

Multiple births

TAMBA (Twins and Multiple Births Association), 2 The Willows,
Gardner Road, Guildford GU1 4PG. Tel: 0870 770 3305.

Multiple sclerosis

Multiple Sclerosis Society of Great Britain and Northern Ireland,
372 Edgeware Road, London NW2 6ND. Tel: 0208 438 0700.

Multiple Sclerosis Resource Centre, 7 Peartree Road, Stanway, Colchester
CO3 5JN. Tel: 01206 505444.

Muscular dystrophy

Muscular Dystrophy Group of Great Britain, 7/11 Prescott Place,
London SW4 6BS. Tel: 0207 720 8055.

Myalgic encephalitis

ME Association, 7 Top Angel, Buckingham Industrial Park, Buckinghamshire
MK18 1TH.

Myasthenia gravis

Myasthenia Gravis Association, Keynes House, Chester Park, Alfreton Road,
Derby DE21 4AS. Tel: 01332 290219.

Myopathy

see Muscular dystrophy

Narcolepsy

Narcolepsy Association (UK), PO Box 3842, Penicuik EH25 8WX.
Tel: 0845 450 0394.

Nursing

Royal College of Nursing, 20 Cavendish Square, London W1M OAB.
Tel: 0207 409 3333.

Osteoporosis

National Osteoporosis Society, PO Box 10, Camerton, Bath BA2 0PJ.
Tel: 01761 471771.

Paget's disease

National Association for the Relief of Paget's Disease, 323 Manchester Road,
Walkden, Worsley, Manchester M28 3HH. Tel: 0161 799 6511.

Paralysis

Spinal Injuries Association, 387–391 Midsummer Boulevard, Milton Keynes
MK9 3HP. Tel: 0845 678 6633.

Spinal Injuries Scotland, Festival Business Centre, 150 Broad Street,
Glasgow G51 1DH. Tel: 0141 314 0056.

Motor Neurone Disease Association, PO Box 246, Northampton NN1 2PR.
Tel: 01604 622269.

Parkinson's disease

Parkinson's Disease Society of the UK, 2215 Vauxhall Bridge Road,
London SW1V 1EJ. Tel: 0207 931 8080.

Phenylketonuria

National Society for Phenylketonuria (UK) Ltd, PO Box 26642, London
N14 4ZF. Tel: 0845 603 9136.

Phobias

National Phobics Society, 339 Stretford Road, Hulme, Manchester M15 4ZY.
Tel: 0870 7700 456.

Psoriasis

National Psoriasis Association, Milton House, 7 Milton Street,
Northampton NN2 7JG. Tel: 01604 711129.

Restricted growth

Restricted Growth Association (RGA), PO Box 4744, Dorchester DT2 9FA. Tel. 01308 898445.

Sickle-cell anaemia

Sickle Cell Society, 54 Station Road, Harlesden, London NW10 4UA. Tel: 0208 961 7795/4006.

Speech disorders

AFASIC (Unlocking Speech and Language), 2nd Floor, 50–52 Great Sutton Street, London EC1N 0DJ. Tel: 0207 378 1200.

Speech therapy

Royal College of Speech and Language Therapists, 2 White Hart Yard, London SE1 1NX. Tel: 0207 378 1200.

Spina bifida

Association for Spina Bifida and Hydrocephalus, ASBAH House, 42 Park Road, Peterborough PE1 2U1. Tel: 01733 555988.

Scottish Spina Bifida Association, 189 Queensferry Road, Edinburgh EH4 2BW. Tel: 0131 332 0743.

Sudden heart death syndrome

Foundation for the Study of Sudden Heart Deaths, Artillery House, 11–19 Artillery Row, London SW1P 1RT. Tel: 0870 787 0885.

Talking books

Calibre, Aylesbury, Bucks HP22 5XQ. Tel: 01296 432339.

Listening Books, 12 Lant Street, London SE1 1QH. Tel: 0207 407 9417.

Tinnitus

see Deafness

Toy libraries

National Association of Toy and Leisure Libraries/Playmatters, 68 Churchway, London NW1 1LT. Tel: 0207 387 9592.

Turner's syndrome

UK Turner Syndrome Society, 12 Irving Quadrant, Hardgate, Clydebank G81 6AZ. Tel: 01389 380 385.

Voluntary organisations

National Council for Voluntary Organisations, Regents Wharf, 8 All Saints Street, London N1 9RL. Tel: 0207 713 6161.

Measurements in medicine

SI units commonly used in medicine

Quantity	SI unit (abbreviation)
Length	Metre (m)
Area	Square metre (m^2)
Volume	Cubic metre (m^3) = 100 litres (L)
Mass	Kilogram (kg)
Amount of substance	Mole (mol)
Energy	Joule (J)
Pressure	Pascal (Pa)
Force	Newton (N)
Time	Second (s)
Frequency	Hertz (Hz)
Power	Watt (w)
Temperature	Degree Celsius (°C)

Multiples and submultiples

Factor	Prefix	Abbreviation
10^6	Mega-	M
10^3	Kilo-	k
10^{-1}	Deci-	d
10^{-2}	Centi-	c
10^{-3}	Milli-	m
10^{-6}	Micro-	
10^{-9}	Nano-	n
10^{-12}	Pico-	p

APPENDIX **12**

International organisations

World Health Organization (WHO)

Founded in 1948, the WHO is a United Nations Agency whose objectives are to attain the highest possible level of health worldwide and to eradicate infectious disease through vaccination programmes.

The organisation is based in Geneva with an office in each of its six regions, usually in the ministry of health.

Its functions include the following:

- setting standards in healthcare

- advocating health policy reform

- working closely with governments in the areas of maternal and child health, populations, planning, nutrition, sanitation, and the supply and distribution of medicines.

Policy is set out at the Annual General Meeting of the World Assembly, which is attended by representatives from member states. The WHO is headed by its director general, who is supported by administrative, technical and medical staff.

The WHO has been successful in the eradication of smallpox, with the last reported case occurring in 1977.

World Medical Association (WMA)

The WMA is an independent confederation of non-governmental professional medical associations from around the world, founded in 1947. The association is non-political and provides a forum for member associations to communicate with each other and to achieve consensus.

The WMA promotes the following:

- high standards of professional medical care and ethics

- professional freedom of physicians thereby facilitating high-calibre medical care.

Since its foundation, and through its declarations, the WMA has developed guidance for doctors, national medical associations, governments and other international bodies. The areas covered include patients' rights, research on humane subjects, torture of prisoners, use and misuse of drugs, family planning and the care of sick and wounded people in times of conflict.

Commonwealth Medical Association (CMA)

The Commonwealth Medical Association is a non-governmental body that has a good working relationship with both the World Health Organization and the health aspects of the United Nations.

The CMA is based in the UK and is subscribed to by a number of national medical associations.

The CMA's main objectives are as follows:

- to strengthen the capacity of national medical associations by collaborating with other health professional associations

- to improve the health status of vulnerable and disadvantaged groups in developing countries.

The main activities of the Association are in the fields of women's, young people's and sexual health. It is also concerned with the ethical and human rights implications of providing health information and services.

Professional organisations relating to complementary medicine

Acupuncture

British Medical Acupuncture Society, Newton House, Newton Lane, Whitley, Warrington WA4 4JA. Tel: 01925 730727.

British Acupuncture Council, Park House, 206–208 Latimer Road, London W10 6RE. Tel: 0208 964 0222.

Alexander technique

Society of Teachers of the Alexander Technique, 20 London House, 266 Fulham Road, London SW10 8EL. Tel: 0207 351 0828.

Aromatherapy

Aromatherapy Organisations Council, 3 Latymer Close, Braybrooke, Market Harborough LE16 9LN. Tel: 01858 434242.

Chiropractic

British Chiropractic Association, 29 Whitley Street, Reading, Berkshire RG2 03G. Tel: 01734 757557.

Chiropractic Patients Association, 8 Centre One, Lysander Way, Old Sarum Park, Salisbury, Wiltshire SP4 6BU. Tel: 01722 415027.

Homeopathy

British Homeopathic Association, 271 Devonshire Street, London WIN 1RJ. Tel: 0207 935 2163.

Faculty of Homeopathy, 2 Powis Place, Great Ormond Street, London WC1N 3HT. Tel: 0207 837 9469.

Hydrotherapy

Chartered Society of Physiotherapists, 14 Bedford Row, London WC1R 4ED. Tel: 0207 306 6666.

Hypnotherapy

British Society of Medical and Dental Hypnosis, 17 Keppel View Road, Kimberworth, Rotherham, Yorkshire S61 2AR. Tel: 01709 554558.

National School of Hypnotherapy and Psychotherapy, The Central Register of Advanced Hypnotherapists, 28 Finsbury Park Road, London N4 2JX. Tel: 0207 359 6991.

Osteopathy

General Council and Register of Osteopaths, 56 London Street, Reading, Berkshire RG1 4SQ. Tel: 01734 576585.

Reflexology

Association of Reflexologists, 27 Old Gloucester Street, London WC1 3XX. Tel: 0870 5673320.

British Reflexology Association, Monks Orchard, Whitbourne, Worcestershire WR6 5RB. Tel: 01886 821207.

The Wanless Report

In 2001, the Chancellor commissioned Derek Wanless, former Chief Executive of the Nat West Bank, to examine demand and cost pressures in the NHS over the next 20 years and recommend the spending needed for a 'publicly funded, comprehensive, high-quality service available on the basis of clinical need and not ability to pay'. The Wanless review team produced an interim report for consultation in November 2001, and published its final report in 2002.

Wanless found that although an ageing population would be an important influence, this would not be the main factor driving up costs. Patients were likely to demand more choice and higher-quality services. Improving information and communication technology would be key to achieving this, while the NHS would have to change its skill mix and ways of working, and enhance the role of primary care.

Wanless concluded that spending would need to rise by between 9% and 11% of GDP in 20 years' time, with the fastest growth before 2008. He warned that 'Both additional resources and radical reform are vital: neither will succeed without the other'.

His figures assume that plans for huge expansion of the workforce are achieved, and that spending on information technology can be doubled and used productively, while the NHS fulfils its commitments on waiting times and National Service Frameworks. If productivity improvement falls short of 2% a year, spending will need to rise to an even higher proportion of GDP.

The Wanless Report endorsed decentralising the NHS, and argued that targets 'should be used with care'. There should be stability and certainty of funding, taking account of local needs without creating perverse incentives. Wanless also called for greater transparency and better understanding of healthcare costs.

Index